Praise for *Patients Beyond Borders*

"The $20 billion-a-year global medical-tourism market finally has a guidebook of its own. With medical tourism now growing at 15 percent annually . . . this tome couldn't be more timely."   —*Travel + Leisure* Magazine

"*Patients Beyond Borders* tells how to plan and budget for medical care abroad and how to find the best doctors and hospitals."   —*AARP Bulletin*

"Woodman suggests a $6,000 rule: if your procedure would cost more than $6,000 in the United States, you would likely save money—possibly more than $1,000—by traveling to a foreign hospital, including all other costs."

—National Public Radio (NPR)

"I have read and am impressed by this book."   —Arthur Frommer

"The bible for the potential surgical traveler."   —Milken Institute

"A must-read for those considering medical tourism."   —ABC News

"*Patients Beyond Borders* is a landmark series of consumer guides to international medical travel that has helped thousands of patients plan successful health journeys abroad."   —*US News & World Report*

What patients are saying about
Patients Beyond Borders

"I spent a lot of time on the Internet trying to research this topic on my own and looking for certain procedures (mainly dental and cosmetic surgery). I wound up getting dental work done in Mexico at a facility reviewed in this book and am happy with my experience. I recommend this book."

—K. Williamson, New Mexico, United States

"I am considering elective surgery, and this was a great compendium of information scattered all over the Internet."

—Amy T., North Carolina, United States

"*Patients Beyond Borders* was my guide through the process of considering, researching, deliberating, and deciding to go abroad for surgery. . . . The book rarely left my side in the months I was considering medical travel."

—Nancy S., North Carolina, United States

"When I went abroad for my surgery, a guide like this would have saved me a lot of time and even more money. Health travel is rewarding, but it can be complicated and it is hard to stay organized. *Patients Beyond Borders* makes planning and taking a trip so much easier."   —Doug S., Wisconsin, United States

"I am a single mom and knew I would be paying out of pocket and wanted someplace safe, so I read [*Patients Beyond Borders*] to help me prepare for my journey."

—Kelly B., Tennessee, United States

Patients Beyond Borders®

Monterrey, Mexico Edition

Everybody's Guide to Affordable, World-Class Healthcare

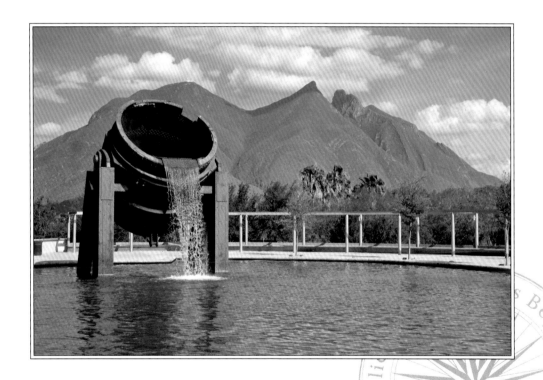

Josef Woodman

HEALTHY TRAVEL MEDIA

patientsbeyondborders.com

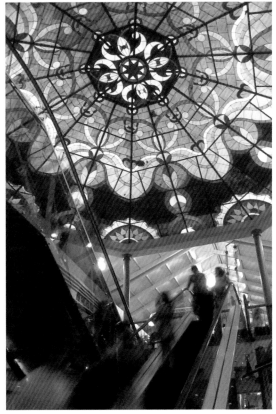

Plaza Mexico, shopping center

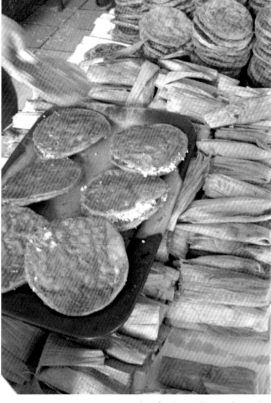

Market fresh tortillas and tamales

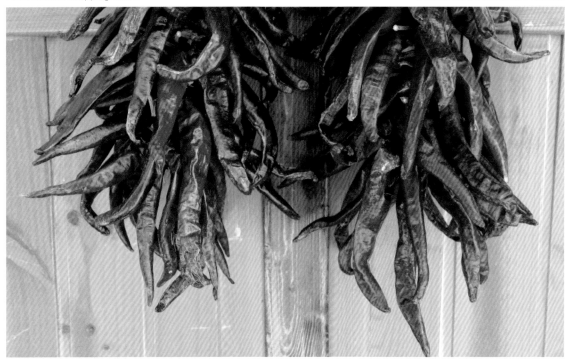

Dried chili peppers, an important ingredient in flavorful Mexican cuisine

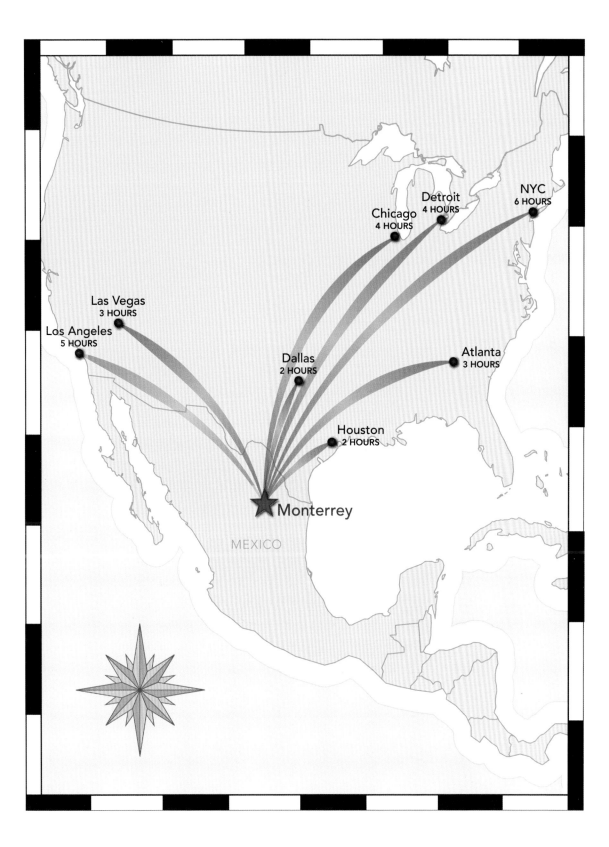

Las Vegas
3 HOURS

Los Angeles
5 HOURS

Chicago
4 HOURS

Detroit
4 HOURS

NYC
6 HOURS

Dallas
2 HOURS

Atlanta
3 HOURS

Houston
2 HOURS

★ Monterrey

MEXICO

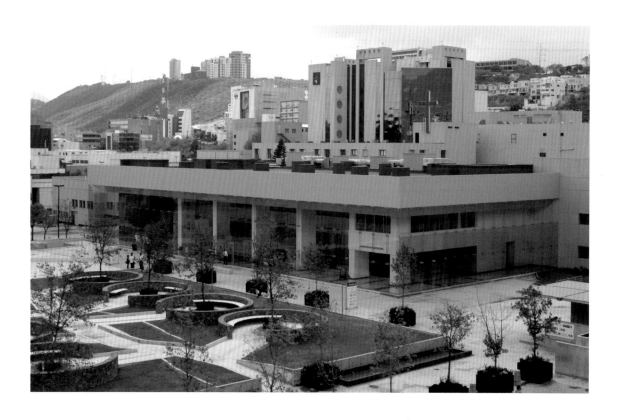

Hospital
San José
Tec de
Monterrey

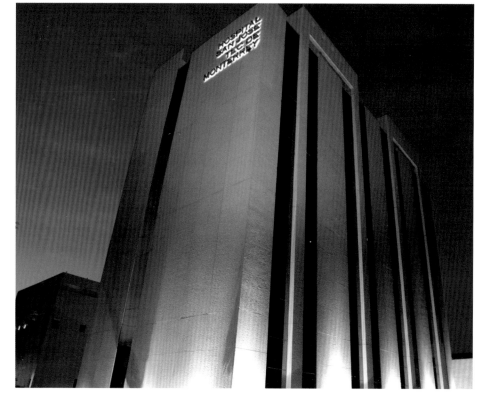

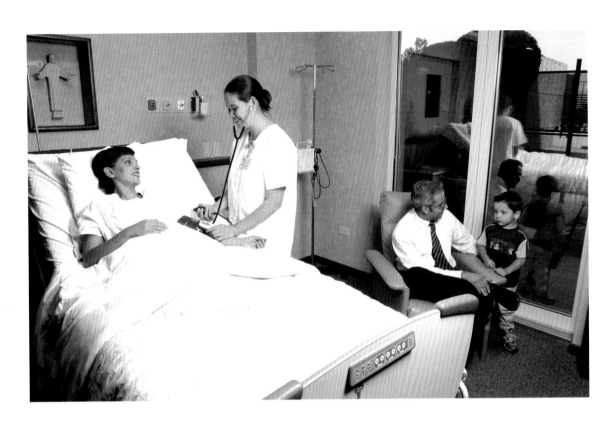

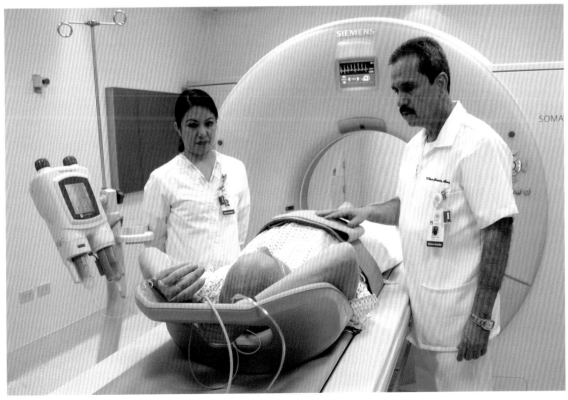

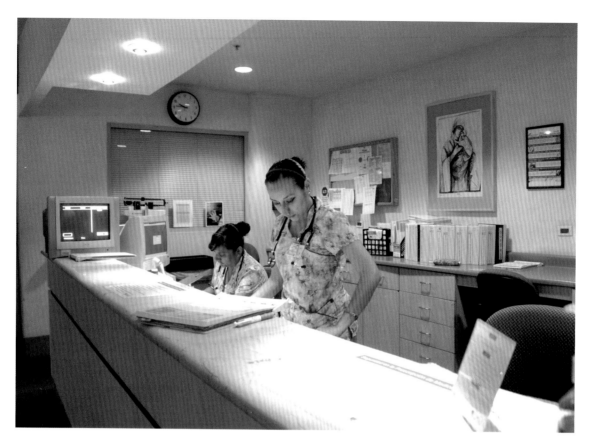

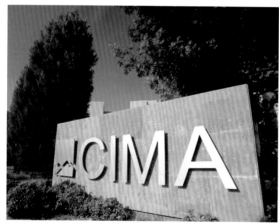

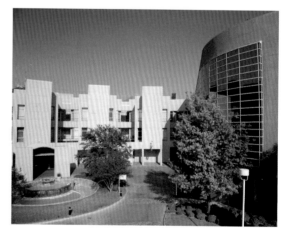

Hospital CIMA Monterrey

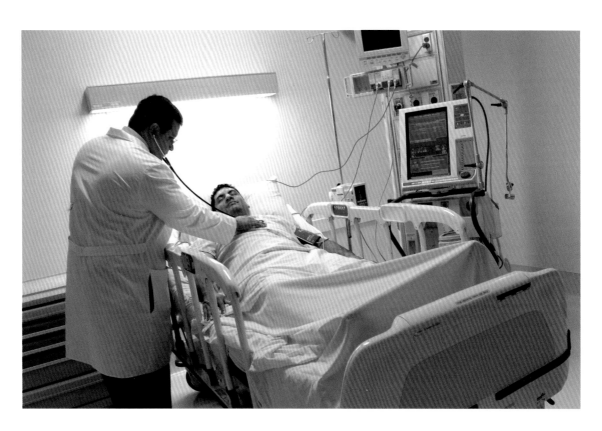

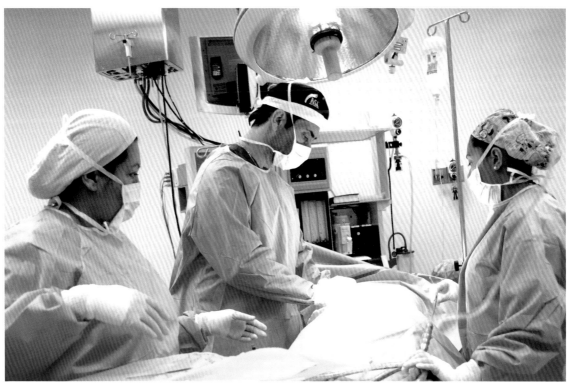

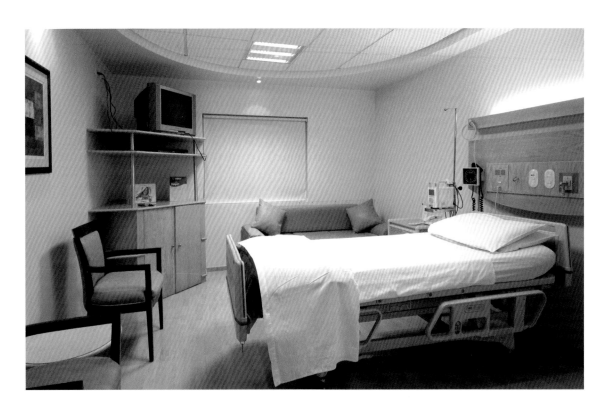

Centro de Ginecología y Obstetricia de Monterrey (Ginequito)

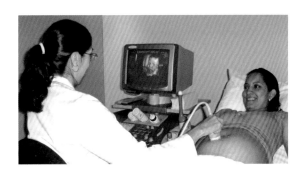

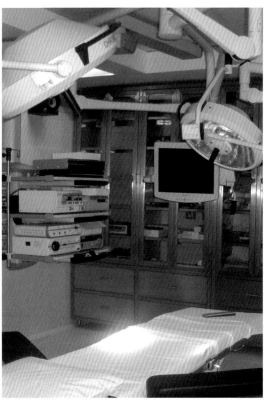

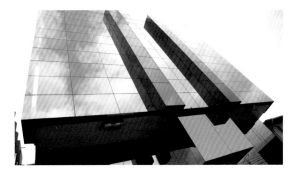

Patients Beyond Borders®

Monterrey, Mexico Edition

Everybody's Guide to Affordable, World-Class Healthcare

Josef Woodman

HEALTHY TRAVEL MEDIA

patientsbeyondborders.com

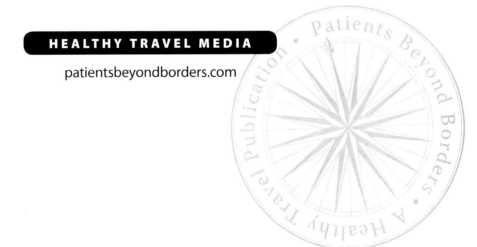

Patients Beyond Borders:
MONTERREY, MEXICO EDITION
Everybody's Guide to Affordable, World-Class Healthcare

Copyright © 2012 by Josef Woodman

ISBN: 978-0-9846095-0-5

COVER ART AND PAGE DESIGN: *Anne Winslow*
EDITORIAL DIRECTION: *Faith Brynie*
DEVELOPMENTAL EDITING: *Jeannette de Beauvoir*
COPYEDITING: *Kate Johnson*
PROOFREADING: *Barbara Resch*
INDEXING: *Madge Walls*
TYPESETTING: *Copperline Book Services*
EBOOK CONVERSION: *BW&A Books*
COMMUNICATIONS: *Judy Orchard*

Healthy Travel Media
P.O. Box 17057
Chapel Hill, NC, UNITED STATES 27516
1 800 883.5740
+1 919 924.0636
info@patientsbeyondborders.com
patientsbeyondborders.com

To All the Dedicated Healthcare Workers
of Monterrey, Mexico

Limits of Liability and Disclaimer of Warranty
Please Read Carefully

This book is intended as a reference guide, not as a medical guide or manual for self-diagnosis or self-treatment. While the intent of *Patients Beyond Borders: Monterrey, Mexico Edition* is to provide useful and informative data, neither the author nor any other party affiliated with this book renders or recommends the use of specific hospitals, clinics, professional services (including physicians and surgeons), third-party agencies, or any other source cited throughout this book.

Patients Beyond Borders: Monterrey, Mexico Edition should not be used as a substitute for advice from a medical professional. The author and publisher expressly disclaim responsibility for any adverse effects that might arise from the information found in *Patients Beyond Borders: Monterrey, Mexico Edition* or any other book, website, or information associated with *Patients Beyond Borders*. Readers who suspect they may have a specific medical problem should consult a physician about any suggestions made in this book.

Hospitals, clinics, or any other treatment institution cited throughout *Patients Beyond Borders: Monterrey, Mexico Edition* are responsible for all treatment provided to patients, including but not limited to surgical, medical, wellness, beauty, and all related queries, opinions, and complications. The author, publisher, editors, and all other parties affiliated with this book are not responsible for same, including any emergency, complication, or medical requirement of whatsoever nature, arising from the patient's treatment due to the patient's present or past illness, or the side effects of drugs or lack of adequate treatment. All pre-treatments, treatments, and post-treatments are the absolute responsibility of the hospital, clinic, or any other treating institution, and/or the treating physician.

ACKNOWLEDGMENTS

EVERY WORTHWHILE PUBLISHED WORK is a group effort. *Patients Beyond Borders: Monterrey, Mexico Edition* is certainly no exception, having grown from the labor of so many able and talented individuals. The people I met during these months of research and production have rewarded me with the unique richness of Mexican hospitality, good humor, and a collaborative spirit so vital to a successful publishing outcome.

I wish to specifically express my gratitude to the many institutions that enthusiastically supported and sponsored this project from the beginning. Monterrey Healthcare City (MHC) played a major role, and I greatly appreciate the early support of Dr. Jesus Horacio Gonzalez Treviño, without whose sustained efforts this project would not have come to fruition. My appreciation also goes to Emilia López-Portillo of MHC for her relentless coordination of all the "moving parts" involved in bringing a book to completion. *Gracias*, Emilia, for taking me to experience firsthand the many wonderful sights of Monterrey—and for introducing me to *cabrito*!

Special thanks to Julio Valdez of the Monterrey Mexico Convention and Visitors Bureau, and to Sergio Eduardo Pérez Zambrano of Agrupimiento Industriales, for their vision and early support.

I am grateful to Dr. Joseph Barcie of CIMA Healthcare and to Sebastián Viramontes of Hospital San José Tec de Monterrey, for their initial contributions to shaping this book's editorial scope. Thanks also to Balbina Lankenau, Cassandra Fuentes, Marcelo García Ayala, Noemí Villanueva López, Dr. Alberto Carillo, Dr. Enrique Chinchilla, and Yolanda Ramirez Cavazos for their collective efforts and provision of critical details.

And thank you to the patients who shared their stories with us. Their voices add a compelling personal touch—and hopefully give an extra sense of comfort to those considering traveling to Monterrey for medical care.

Finally, a heartfelt note of appreciation to the editors, proofreaders, designers, and indexer who made the *Monterrey, Mexico Edition* possible. Special thanks to Jeannette de Beauvoir and Faith Brynie, who crafted the manuscript; to Kate Johnson, who copyedited and polished these pages; and to Anne Winslow and Nicki Florence, for their meticulous attention to detail and design.

Josef Woodman
Chapel Hill NC
January 2012

Contents

Preface

EVERY TIME I GO TO MONTERREY I am amazed by the changes I see. The city is not only a center of excellence for a number of different industries but also a constantly evolving cosmopolitan area, and I'm always glad to look in and see what's new. Monterrey's most affluent districts rival Beverly Hills, while other parts remind visitors of European capitals. It's an industrial hub: if you've ever used printer cartridges, turned on an air conditioner, had a drink from a watercooler, or depended on a car battery, chances are that you used components made in Monterrey. What's more, Monterrey's population of 4 million is the most educated in Mexico, and there are more colleges, universities, and institutes of technology per capita than anywhere else in Mexico.

All that, and the best healthcare in the country. While in the past Mexico was known mainly for dentistry and cosmetic surgery, Monterrey now offers nearly every imaginable procedure—from knee replacement to weight loss surgery, from cardiovascular surgery to oncology—all in American-accredited facilities with board-certified practitioners. With Monterrey's medical schools supporting teaching hospitals, medical travelers also get the most up-to-date treatments and the benefit of the latest in medical research.

Growth in Monterrey is clearly continuing. Of the nine Joint Commission International (JCI)–accredited hospitals in Mexico, four are in Monterrey; in addition, the city is home to a number of private international specialty hospitals and clinics. One of the leading hospitals has just opened a new 520-bed facility. Monterrey's commitment to healthcare includes three first-rate medical schools: Tecnológico de Monterrey, Universidad de Monterrey, and the new Universidad Autónoma de Nuevo León. Furthermore, a number of Monterrey's hospitals and universities enjoy affiliations and working partnerships with prestigious US hospitals such as Johns Hopkins.

These days, medical travelers sometimes worry about their safety in a foreign country. Despite the social and political travails Mexico is currently experiencing, Monterrey is in a far better position to safely serve the medical traveler than are the more infamous towns along the border. Furthermore, your experience in Monterrey will be as protected as you wish it to be. If you make arrangements through your hospital or a medical travel agent, you'll be picked up from the airport and taken to your hotel; in fact, all transportation to and from your hotel will probably be provided for you.

Aside from your hospital stay, you're free to explore a city that has as many tourist attractions as it does medical ones—along with some of the best food I've eaten anywhere. During your pre-treatment or recovery time, treat yourself to a look around. The Parque Fundidora is truly remarkable, and Monterrey's "old city" is close to the city center and a lot of fun to walk around. Try to see Monterrey from high up—either Obispado or Chipinque—and dine on the local specialty, *cabrito* (baby goat), at the renowned El Rey del Cabrito.

Today, Monterrey can be welcomed into the ranks of the leading global healthcare venues. The city offers medical, research, and industrial infrastructure to its hospitals and clinics, and I can say with confidence that Monterrey is an international rising star with a bright and optimistic future.

Josef Woodman
January 2012

Introduction

IF YOU'RE HOLDING THIS COPY of *Patients Beyond Borders: Monterrey, Mexico Edition* in your hands, you probably already know that you need a medical procedure, and perhaps you are considering an affordable, trustworthy alternative to care in your own country. As you can see, this is a specialty volume in the *Patients Beyond Borders* series, profiling Monterrey, Mexico, as a healthcare destination. It is intended for those who already have (more or less) a diagnosis and already know (more or less) what treatment they need.

This edition doesn't provide the breadth of general information about international medical travel that you'll find in our larger book, *Patients Beyond Borders: Everybody's Guide to Affordable, World-Class Healthcare*, now in its Third Edition. Instead, this volume first offers an overview of the questions you need to answer before you commit to medical travel; then, most of its pages are devoted to describing the best places in Monterrey to find excellent treatment and care. This book also contains information on health travel agents who can help you make the necessary arrangements in Monterrey at a reasonable price.

Patients Beyond Borders: Monterrey, Mexico Edition isn't a guide to medical diagnosis and treatment, nor does it provide medical advice on specific treatments or caregiver referrals. Your condition, diagnosis, treatment options, and travel preferences are unique, and only you—in consultation with your physician and loved ones—can determine the best course of action. Should you decide to go to Monterrey for treatment, we provide a wealth of resources and tools to help you become an informed medical traveler, so you can have the best possible travel experience and treatment your money can buy.

The Phenomenon of Medical Travel

My research, including countless interviews, has convinced me that with diligence, perseverance, and good information, patients considering traveling to Monterrey or any other place for healthcare indeed have legitimate, safe choices, not to mention an opportunity to save thousands of dollars over the same treatment in their home country. Depending upon the country and type of treatment, uninsured and underinsured patients, as well as those seeking elective care, can save 50–70 percent of the cost of treatment in their home country. For example, a knee replacement that costs $34,000 in the US may cost $10,000 in Monterrey.

Estimated Costs in US Dollars	Heart Bypass	Hip Replacement	Facelift	Gastric Bypass	Robotic-Assisted Prostatectomy
Monterrey, Mexico*	$36,000	$14,400	$5,500	$12,000	$24,700
United States**	$88,000	$33,000	$11,000	$25,000	$49,000

*Monterrey costs are averages based on data reported as of 2010.

**US costs vary widely depending on location, materials and equipment, and individual requirements. Rates are averages and reflect discounts available to uninsured patients.

But cost savings are the not the only reason to travel for healthcare. Others include:

Better quality care. Veteran health travelers know that facilities, instrumentation, and customer service in treatment centers abroad often equal or exceed those found in their own country.

Excluded treatments. Many people don't have health insurance. Even if you do, your policy may exclude a variety of conditions and treatments. You, the policyholder, must pay these expenses out of pocket, so having the procedure in a place where it's more affordable makes economic sense.

Specialty treatments. Some procedures not available in your home country are available abroad. Some procedures that are widely practiced in certain parts of the world have not yet been approved in others, or they have been approved so recently that their availability remains spotty.

Shorter waiting periods. For decades, thousands of Canadian and British subscribers to universal, "free" healthcare plans have endured long waits for established procedures. Patients living in other countries with socialized medicine are beginning to experience longer waits as well. Some patients figure it's better to pay out of pocket to get out of pain or halt a deteriorating condition than to suffer the anxiety and frustration of waiting.

More "inpatient-friendly." Health insurance companies apply significant pressure on hospitals to move patients out of those costly beds as quickly as possible, sometimes before they are ready. In Monterrey and many other medical travel destinations, care is taken to ensure that patients are discharged only at the appropriate time and no sooner. Furthermore, staff-to-patient ratios are usually higher abroad, while hospital-borne infection rates are often lower.

The lure of the new and different. Although traveling abroad for medical care can often be challenging, many patients welcome the chance to blaze a trail, and they find the hospitality and creature comforts often offered abroad to be a welcome relief from the sterile, impersonal hospital environments so frequently encountered at home.

How to Use This Book

Before you dive into **Part Two**, please review the checklists and sidebars in **Part One, "Reminders for the Savvy, Informed Medical Traveler."** A shortened version of the more complete information in the international *Patients Beyond Borders: Third Edition*, it gives you some of the tools you'll need to do your research and make an informed decision. You'll find the following in Part One:

Dos and Don'ts for the Smart Health Traveler
Patients Beyond Borders **Budget Planner**
Checklists for Health Travel
    Checklist 1: Should I Consult a Health Travel Planner?
    Checklist 2: What Do I Need to Do Ahead of Time?
    Checklist 3: What Should I Pack?
    Checklist 4: What Do I Do After My Procedure?
    Checklist 5: What Does My Travel Companion Need to Do?

Part Two, "Monterrey, Mexico: A Prime Destination for the Medical Traveler," provides a brief overview of healthcare in Monterrey today and profiles prominent healthcare facilities as well as several health travel agencies that serve medical travelers to Monterrey. Each entry provides contact information along with a rundown on available services and history of care.

Part Three, "Traveling in Monterrey, Mexico," provides details on everything from passports to pastimes—basic, practical information you'll need to plan your trip. It also describes a number of the sights and experiences to be enjoyed in Monterrey and offers advice on staying safe and staying well.

Part Four, "Resources and References," offers additional sources of travel information and helpful links.

As you work your way through decision-making and subsequent planning, remember that you're following in the footsteps of millions of health travelers who have made the journey before you. The vast majority have returned home successfully treated, with money to spare in their savings accounts. Still, the process—particularly in the early planning—can be daunting, frustrating, and even a little scary. Every health traveler I've interviewed experienced "the Big Fear" at one time or another. Healthcare abroad is not for everyone, and part of being a smart consumer is evaluating all the impartial data available before making an informed decision. If you accomplish that in reading *Patients Beyond Borders: Monterrey, Mexico Edition*, I've achieved my goal. Let's get started.

Part One

Reminders for the Savvy, Informed Medical Traveler

Much of the advice in Part One is covered in greater detail in the international *Patients Beyond Borders: Third Edition*. Consider the following three sections a capsule summary of essential information, sprinkled with practical advice that will help reduce the number of inevitable "gotchas" that health travelers encounter. You may want your travel companion or family members to read this section, along with the book's Introduction, so they can gain a better understanding of medical travel.

Dos and Don'ts
for the Smart Health Traveler

———— — ———— — ———— — ———— — ———— — ————

Before Your Trip

Do plan ahead.

The farther in advance you plan, the more likely you are to get the best doctors, the lowest airfares, and the best availability and rates on Monterrey hotels, particularly if you'll be traveling at peak tourist season (July through September). If possible, begin planning at least three months prior to your expected departure date. If you're concerned about having to change plans, *do* be sure to confirm cancellation policies with airlines, hotels, and travel agents.

Do be sure about your diagnosis and treatment needs.

The more you know about the treatment you're seeking, the easier your search for a physician will be. *Do* work closely with your local doctor or medical specialist, and make sure you obtain exact recommendations—in writing, if possible. If you lack confidence in your doctor's diagnosis or treatment plan, seek a second opinion.

_Do_ research your in-country doctor thoroughly.
This is the most important step of all. When you've narrowed your search to two or three physicians, invest some time and money in personal telephone interviews, either directly with your candidate doctors or through your health travel planning agency. _Don't_ be afraid to ask questions, lots of them, until you feel comfortable that you have chosen a competent physician.

Don't rely completely on the internet for your research.
While it's okay to use the web for your initial research, _don't_ assume that sponsored websites offer complete and accurate information. Cross-check your online findings against referrals, articles in leading newspapers and magazines, word of mouth, and your health travel agent.

_Do_ consider traveling with a companion.
Many health travelers say they wouldn't go without a close friend or family member by their side. Your travel companion can help you every step of the way. With luck, your companion may even enjoy the trip!

_Do_ consider engaging a good health travel planner.
Even the most intrepid, adventurous medical traveler will benefit from the knowledge, experience, and in-country support these professionals can bring to any health journey. _Do_ thoroughly research an agent before plunking down your deposit.

_Do_ get it in writing.
Cost estimates, appointments, recommendations, opinions, second opinions, airline and hotel arrangements—get as much as you can in writing, and _do_ be sure to take all documentation with you on the plane. Email is fine, as long as you retain a written record of your key transactions. The more you get in writing, the less chance of a misunderstanding.

_Do_ insist on using a language you understand.

As much as many of us would like to have a better command of another language, the time to brush up on your Spanish is most definitely _not_ when negotiating medical care in Monterrey. Establishing comfortable, reliable communication with your key contacts is paramount to your success as a health traveler.

Don't plan your trip too tightly.

A missed consultation or an extra two days of recovery in Monterrey can mean expensive rescheduling with airlines. A good rule of thumb is to add an extra day for every five days you anticipate for consultation, treatment, and recovery.

_Do_ alert your bank and credit card companies.

Contact your bank and credit card companies _prior to your trip._ Inform them of your travel dates and where you will be. If you plan to use a credit card for large amounts, alert the company in advance, and reconfirm your credit limits to avoid card cancellation or unexpected rejections.

_Do_ learn a little about your destination.

Once you've decided on Monterrey or any other health travel destination, spend a little time getting to know something about its history and geography. Buy or borrow a couple of travel guides. Read a local newspaper. Your hosts will appreciate your knowledge and interest.

_Do_ inform your local doctors before you leave.

Preserve a good working relationship with your family physician and local specialists. Although they may not particularly like your traveling overseas for medical care, most doctors will respect your decision. Your local healthcare providers need to know what you're doing, so they can continue your care and treatment once you return home.

While in Monterrey

Don't be too adventurous with local cuisine.

Spicy pork fajitas! Local tequila! Camerones a la diabla! One sure way to get your treatment off to a bad start is to enter your clinic with even a mild case of stomach upset due to a change in drink or diet. Prior to treatment, avoid rich, spicy foods and exotic drinks. Bottled water is safest for your stomach. During any inpatient stay, *don't* be afraid to ask the hospital's dietician for a menu that's easy on your digestion.

Don't scrimp on lodging.

Unless your finances absolutely demand it, avoid hotels and other accommodations in the "budget" category. You *don't* want to end up in uncomfortable surroundings when you're recuperating from major surgery. On the other hand, you should be able to find a good hotel in Monterrey in a price range that suits you. Ask your hospital or health travel agent for a recommendation.

Don't stay too far from your treatment center.

When booking hotel accommodations for you and your companion, make sure the hospital or doctor's office is nearby. Staff members at your destination hospital can advise you on suitable lodging. (Part Three provides information on lodgings near major hospitals in Monterrey.)

Don't settle for second best in treatment options.

While you can cut corners on airfare, lodging, and transportation, always insist on the very best healthcare your money can buy. Focus on quality, not just price.

Do befriend the staff.

Nurses, nurse's aides, paramedics, receptionists, clerks, and even maintenance people are vital members of your health team! Take the time to chat with them, learn their names, inquire about their families, and perhaps proffer a small gift. Above all, treat the staff with deference and respect. When you're ready to leave the hospital, a sincere thank-you note makes a great farewell.

Going Home

Don't return home too soon.

After an airplane flight to Monterrey, multiple consultations with physicians and staff, and a painful and disorienting medical procedure, you might feel ready to jump on the first flight home. That's understandable but not advisable. Your body needs time to recuperate, and your in-country physician needs to track your recovery progress. As you plan your trip, ask your physician how much recovery time is advised for your particular treatment—then add a few extra days, just to be safe. You can always see some of Monterrey's wonderful sights during your extra days, if you feel up to it!

Do set aside some of your medical travel savings for a vacation.

You and your companion deserve it! If you're not able to take leisure time during your medical trip to Monterrey, then set aside a little money for some time off after you return home, even if it's only a weekend getaway.

Do get all your paperwork before leaving the country.

Get copies of everything. No matter how eager you are to get well and get home, make sure you have full documentation on your procedure(s), treatment(s), and followup. Get receipts for everything.

Above All, Trust Your Intuition

Your courage and good judgment have set you on the path to medical travel. Rely on your instincts. If, for example, you feel uncomfortable with your in-country consultation, switch doctors. If you get a queasy feeling about extra or uncharted costs, don't be afraid to question them. Millions of health travelers have beaten a well-worn path abroad, using good information and common sense. You can, too! Safe travels!

Ten "Must-Ask" Questions for Your Candidate Physician

Make the following initial inquiries, either of your health travel agent or the physician(s) you're interviewing:

1. *What are your credentials? Where did you receive your medical degree? Where was your internship? What types of continuing education workshops have you attended recently?* The right international physician either has credentials posted on the web or will be happy to email you a complete résumé.

2. *How many patients do you see each month?* Hopefully, it's more than 50 and less than 500. The physician who says "I don't know" should make you suspicious. Doctors should be in touch with their customer base and have such information readily available.

3. *To what associations do you belong?* Any worthwhile physician or surgeon is a member of at least one medical association, and many Monterrey doctors and facilities have sister offices in the US. Your practitioner should be keeping good company with others in the field.

4. *How many patients have you treated who have had my condition?* There's safety in numbers, and you'll want to know them. Find out how many procedures your intended hospital has performed. Ask how many of your specific treatments for your specific condition your candidate doctor has personally conducted.

5. *What are the fees for your initial consultation?* Answers will vary, and you should compare prices to those of other physicians you interview.

6. *May I call you on your mobile phone before, during, and after treatment?* Most international physicians stay in close, direct contact with their patients, and mobile phones are their tools of choice.

7. *What medical and personal health records do you need to assess my condition and treatment needs?* Most physicians require at least the basics: recent notes and recommendations from consultations with your local physician or specialist(s), x-rays or scans directly related to your condition, perhaps a medical history, and other health records. Be wary of the physician who requires no personal paperwork.

8. *Do you practice alone, or with others in a clinic or hospital?* Look for a physician who practices among a group of certified professionals with a broad range of related skills.

For surgery:

9. *Do you do the surgery yourself, or do you have assistants do the surgery?* This is one area where delegation isn't desirable. You want assurance that your procedure won't be performed by your practitioner's protégé.

10. *Are you the physician who oversees my entire treatment, including pre-surgery, surgery, prescriptions, physical therapy recommendations, and post-surgery checkups?* For larger surgical procedures, you want the designated team captain. While that's usually the surgeon, check to make sure. ■

Patients Beyond Borders
Budget Planner

To derive an estimate of your health travel costs and savings, we suggest you use the *"Patients Beyond Borders* Budget Planner" in this section. As you plan, fill in the blanks that apply to you, and you'll arrive at a rough estimate of your costs—and your savings. (You'll find more details in the international *Patients Beyond Borders: Third Edition.*)

The $6,000 Rule

A good monetary barometer of whether your medical trip is financially worthwhile is the *Patients Beyond Borders* "$6,000 Rule": If your total quote for local treatment (including consultations, procedures, and hospital stay) is US$6,000 or more, you'll probably save money by traveling abroad for your care. If it's less than US$6,000, you're likely better off having your treatment at home.

The application of this rule varies, of course, depending on your financial position and lifestyle preferences. For some, a small savings might offset the hassles of travel. For others who might be traveling anyway, savings considerations are fuzzier.

Patients Beyond Borders Budget Planner

Item	Cost	Comment
IN MONTERREY		
Passport/Visa		
Rush charges, if any:		
Treatment Estimate		
Procedure:		
Hospital room, if extra:		Including facility and physician fees
Lab work, x-rays, if extra:		
Additional consultations:		
Medication, if extra:		
Tips/gifts for staff:		
Other:		
Post-Treatment		
Recuperation lodging:		Hospital room or hotel
Physical therapy:		
Prescriptions:		
Concierge services:		Optional
Other:		
Airfare		
You:		
Your companion:		
Other travelers:		
Airport fees:		Baggage and parking
Other:		

Patients Beyond Borders Budget Planner (*continued*)

Item	Cost	Comment
Room and Board		
Hotel:		
Food:		
Taxis, buses, limos:		
Entertainment/sightseeing:		
Other:		
"While You're Away" Costs		
Pet sitter/house sitter:		
Other:		
Other:		
IN MONTERREY SUBTOTAL		
HOMETOWN		
Procedure:		Including facility and physician fees
Lab work, x-rays:		
Hospital room:		
Additional consultations:		
Physical therapy:		
Prescriptions:		
Other:		
HOMETOWN SUBTOTAL		
TOTAL SAVINGS:		Subtract In Monterrey Subtotal from Hometown Subtotal

Patients Beyond Borders Sample Budget Planner

Item	Cost	Comment
IN MONTERREY		
Passport/Visa	$200.00	
Rush charges, if any:		
Treatment Estimate		
Procedure:	$9,000.00	
Hospital room, if extra:		Including facility and physician fees
Lab work, x-rays, if extra:	$45.00	
Additional consultations:	$200.00	
Medication, if extra:		
Tips/gifts for staff:	$100.00	
Other:		
Post-Treatment		
Recuperation lodging:	$1,100.00	Hospital room or hotel
Physical therapy:	$65.00	
Prescriptions:	$65.00	
Concierge services:	$300.00	Optional
Other:		
Airfare		
You:	$880.00	
Your companion:	$880.00	
Other travelers:		
Airport fees:	$50.00	Baggage and parking
Other:		

Patients Beyond Borders Sample Budget Planner (*continued*)

Item	Cost	Comment
Room and Board		
Hotel:	$1,500.00	
Food:	$650.00	
Taxis, buses, limos:	$200.00	
Entertainment/sightseeing:	$500.00	
Other:		
"While You're Away" Costs		
Pet sitter/house sitter:	$300.00	
Other:		
Other:		
IN MONTERREY SUBTOTAL	$16,035.00	
HOMETOWN		
Procedure:	$55,000.00	Including facility and physician fees
Lab work, x-rays:	$375.00	
Hospital room:	$4,400.00	
Additional consultations:	$1,200.00	
Physical therapy:	$400.00	
Prescriptions:	$500.00	
Other:		
HOMETOWN SUBTOTAL	$61,875.00	
TOTAL SAVINGS:	$45,840.00	Subtract In Monterrey Subtotal
		from Hometown Subtotal

Will My Health Insurance Cover My Overseas Medical Expenses?

As of this writing, it's possible, but not probable. While the largest employers and healthcare insurers—not to mention ever-vocal politicians—struggle with new models of coverage, most plans do not yet cover the costs of obtaining treatment abroad. Yet, with healthcare costs threatening to literally bust some Western economies, pressures for change are mounting. Recognizing that the globalization of healthcare is now a reality—and that developed countries are falling behind—insurers, employers, and hospitals are beginning to form partnerships with payers and providers abroad. By the time you read this book, large insurers may already be offering coverage (albeit limited) across borders. Check with your insurer for the latest on your coverage abroad.

Can I Sue?

For better or worse, many countries do not share the Western attitude toward personal and institutional liability. A full discussion of the reasons lies outside the scope of this book. Here's a good rule of thumb: if legal recourse is a primary concern in making your health travel decision, you probably shouldn't head abroad for medical treatment.

If, however, you experience severe complications and do not receive the followup care you think you need or deserve, then you may want to consider legal action. It can be done, although the process can be complex—you'll need some serious professional help.

The good news is that informed patients can take preventive measures to protect themselves before they travel abroad for care, so they do not end up in the hands of imperfect healthcare insurance and judicial systems. Furthermore, foreign hospitals are eager to prove that the quality of their surgeons and facilities rivals or even exceeds that found elsewhere. They understand that the publicity associated with even one bad outcome could quickly end the growing flow of health travelers. They'll go a long way to prevent a negative result.

Your Medical Trip May Be Tax-Deductible

Depending on the country you live in, your medical travel expenses may be tax-deductible. In the US, for example, depending on your income level and treatment cost, some or most of your health journey can be itemized as a deduction from your adjusted gross income. If the total amounts to more than 7.5 percent of adjusted gross income, the Internal Revenue Service (IRS) allows US citizens to deduct the remainder of those expenses. Examples of typical tax-deductible items include

- any treatment normally covered by a health insurance plan
- transportation expenses, including air, train, boat, or road travel
- lodging and meals for duration of treatment
- recovery hotels, surgical retreats, and recuperation resorts

If you are planning to take a tax deduction, ask for letters and other documentation from your in-country healthcare provider, particularly any recommendations made for outside lodging, special diets, and other services. For more information, US citizens can go to irs.gov or call 1 800 829.1040. Medical travelers from other countries should check their government's tax policies. It's always a good idea to consult a competent tax advisor with questions or concerns.

Checklists for Health Travel

The five checklists that follow will remind you of some important issues you need to consider in planning your health travel. If you desire additional information about traveling abroad for treatment, you may want to buy or borrow a copy of the international *Patients Beyond Borders: Third Edition*, which contains more information and additional checklists.

Checklist 1: *Should I Consult a Health Travel Planner?*

Health travel planners answer to many names: brokers, facilitators, agents, expeditors. Throughout this book, we use the phrase "health travel planner" or "health travel agent" to mean any agency or representative who specializes in helping patients obtain medical treatment abroad. Before engaging the services of a health travel agent, ask yourself these questions:

Whether to use a health travel planner	Yes	No	Not Sure
Will a health travel planner save me time?			
Am I willing to pay for the convenience of a health travel planner's services?			
Will I feel more confident about health travel if I use the services of an agency?			
Does the agent I'm considering have the knowledge and experience I need?			
Does this planner have a track record of successful service to the health traveler?			
Does this agent speak my language well enough for us to converse comfortably?			
Can I get at least two recommendations or letters of reference from former clients of this agency? Have I checked these references?			
Can I get at least two recommendations or letters of reference from treatment centers that work with this agency? Have I checked these references?			
Can this agency give me complete information about possible destinations and options for my procedure?			
Will this agent put me in touch with one or more treatment centers and physicians?			
Will this agent work collaboratively to help me choose the best treatment option?			
Is this agent responsive to my questions and concerns?			
Does the service package this agent is offering meet my needs?			
Does this agent have longstanding affiliations with in-country treatment centers and practitioners?			

Whether to use a health travel planner	Yes	No	Not Sure
Has this planner negotiated better-than-retail rates with hospitals, clinics, physicians, hotels, and (perhaps) airlines?			
Can this agent save me money on other in-country costs, such as airport pickup and dropoff or transportation to my clinic?			
Can this agent provide personal assistance and support in my destination country?			
Is this planner willing to work within the constraints of my budget?			
Do I know (and have in writing) the exact costs for this agency's services?			
Do I have a suitable contract or letter of agreement with this agency?			
Do I feel comfortable with this agency? Have we built a sense of trust?			

Of all the services a health travel planner offers, the most important are related to your treatment. Start your dialogue by asking the fundamental questions: Do you know the best doctors? Have you met personally with your preferred physicians and visited their clinics? Can you give me their credentials and background information? What about accommodations? Do you provide transportation to and from the airport? To and from the treatment center? If an agent is knowledgeable and capable with these details, the rest of the planning usually takes care of itself.

Checklist 2: *What Do I Need to Do Ahead of Time?*

This checklist covers some of the planning you'll need to do to become a fully prepared and informed global patient.

Have I completed these planning steps?	Yes	No
Engaged the services of a health travel planner (if desired — see Checklist 1)		
Obtained a second opinion — or a third if necessary — on diagnosis and treatment options		
Considered a range of treatment options and discussed each option with potential providers		
Reviewed the various hospitals, clinics, specialties, and treatments available to select an appropriate destination (see Part Two)		
Chosen a reliable, fun travel companion		
Obtained and reviewed the professional credentials of two or more physicians or surgeons (see "Ten 'Must-Ask' Questions for Your Candidate Physician" on page 8)		
Selected the best physician or surgeon for the treatment I need		
Researched the history and accreditation of the hospital or clinic (see "The What and Why of JCI" on page 23)		
Checked for the affiliations and partnerships of the hospital or clinic		
Learned about the number of surgeries performed in the hospital or clinic (generally, the more the better)		
Learned about success rates (these are usually calculated as a ratio of successful operations to the overall number of operations performed)		
Gathered and sent all medical records and diagnostic information that my physician or surgeon needs to plan my treatment		
Prearranged travel, accommodations, recovery, and leisure activities (if desired)		
Prearranged amenities, such as concierge services in-country or wheelchair services on the return trip		
Packed the essentials (see Checklist 3)		
Double-checked everything — then checked again		

The What and Why of JCI

When you walk into a hospital or clinic in the US and many other Western countries, chances are good that it's accredited, meaning that it's in compliance with standards and "good practices" set by an independent accreditation agency. In the US, by far the largest and most respected accreditation agency is the Joint Commission. The commission casts a wide net of evaluation for hospitals, clinics, home healthcare, ambulatory services, and a host of other healthcare facilities and services throughout the US.

Responding to a global demand for accreditation standards, in 1999 the Joint Commission launched JCI, its international affiliate accreditation agency. In order to be accredited, an international healthcare provider must meet the rigorous standards set forth by JCI. At this writing, more than 400 hospitals, laboratories, and special programs outside the US have been JCI-approved, with more coming on board each month.

Although JCI accreditation is not essential, it's an important new benchmark and the only medically oriented seal of approval for international hospitals and clinics. Learning that your treatment center is JCI-approved lends comfort to the process, and the remainder of your searching and checking need not be as rigorous. However, many excellent hospitals, while not JCI-approved, have received local accreditation at the same levels as the world's best treatment centers.

JCI's website carries far more information than you'll ever want to explore on accreditation standards and procedures. View JCI's current roster of accredited hospitals abroad at jointcommissioninternational.org. ■

Checklist 3: *What Should I Pack?*

You've likely heard the cardinal rule of international travel: pack light. Less to carry means less to lose. Don't worry if you leave behind some basic item such as shampoo or a comb; you can always pick it up at your destination. That said, this checklist covers the items you absolutely, positively shouldn't forget—and make sure you carry these things in your carry-on bag. A prescription or passport lost in checked luggage could spell disaster.

Is this item packed in my carry-on bag?	Yes	No
Passport		
Visa (if required)		
Travel itinerary		
Airline tickets or eticket confirmations		
Driver's license or valid picture ID (in addition to passport)		
Health insurance card(s) or policy		
ATM card or traveler's checks		
Credit card(s)		
Enough cash for airport fees and local transportation upon arrival		
Immunization record		
Prescription medications		
Hard-to-find over-the-counter drugs		
Medical records, current x-rays/scans, consultations, and treatment notes		
All financial agreements and hard copies of email correspondence		
Phone and fax numbers, mailing addresses, and email addresses of people I need or want to contact in-country		
Phone and fax numbers, mailing addresses, and email addresses of people I need or want to contact back home		
Travel journal for notes, expense records, and receipts		

Continuity of Care

Continuity of care can be a challenge for patients who travel for medical procedures. Excellent communication is critical to the success of your treatment—both with your hometown doctor and your international healthcare team. Many hospitals offer an international patient services center with medically knowledgeable staff fluent in English and other languages.

Make sure you take full advantage of this resource and work with them to fully coordinate your appointments and healthcare plan *before* you schedule your travel. Make sure, also, that you work with them to establish communication between your primary (local) doctor and your in-country medical team. Early communication with both parties can ensure better followup care after you return home.

Current Medical Records

Once you have established contact with your selected facility's international patient center, work with them to make sure your in-country physician will have access to your most current medical records, including up-to-date laboratory tests, x-rays, or scans. Medical records are most often transmitted in two ways: as paper copies or disks by postal service, or as electronic documents via a secure online service.

Collaboration Among Doctors

Transferring your medical records may get your local doctor communicating directly with your in-country physician for the first time. The next collaboration should occur after your treatment or your surgery. Work with the international patient center to make sure your local physician is notified of the details of the surgery and the aftercare protocol. Once you return home and are again under the care of your local physician, this collaboration and consultation should continue until you are released from care with a clean bill of health.

Complete Documentation

Too often, patients return home lacking the complete documentation their local physician needs to oversee ongoing care. The absence of information compromises the physician's effectiveness and threatens the patient's health. Make sure you get complete records before you return home. Also make sure to keep your local physician involved from the first day. ■

CHAPTER THREE

Checklist 4: *What Do I Do After My Procedure?*

Coping with post-surgery discomfort is difficult enough when you're close to home. Lying for long hours in a hospital bed, far away from family— that's often the darkest time for a health traveler. Knowledge is the best antidote to needless worry. As with pre-surgery preparation, ask lots of questions about post-surgery discomforts *before* heading into the operating room. Be sure to ask doctors and nurses about what kinds of discomforts to expect following your specific procedure.

If your discomfort or pain becomes acute, bleeding is persistent, or you suspect a growing infection, you may be experiencing a complication that is more serious than mere discomfort and requires immediate attention. Contact your physician without delay.

This checklist will help you make the most of your post-treatment period and know when it's appropriate to seek medical assistance.

Post-procedure preparations and followup	Yes	No	Not Sure
Have I received all my doctor's instructions for my post-treatment care and recovery? Do I understand them all?			
Am I following all of my physician's instructions *to the letter*?			
Do I know what post-treatment signs and symptoms are normal?			
Do I know what post-treatment signs and symptoms indicate a need for prompt medical attention?			
Do I have copies of all my medical and treatment records, including x-rays/scans, photographs, blood test results, prescriptions, and others?			
Do I have itemized receipts for all the bills I have paid?			
Do I have itemized bills for all the costs I have not yet paid?			
Do I have completed insurance claim forms (if applicable)?			
Have I allotted ample time for recovery?			
Do I know how to prevent blood clots in the legs after surgery and on the airplane?			
Do I know what followup treatment I will need when I return home, including physical therapy?			
Have I let my family know what help I will need when I return home?			

Post-procedure preparations and followup	Yes	No	Not Sure
Have I checked in with my local doctor to share information about the procedure I had and my post-treatment care needs?			
Am I staying mentally, physically, and socially active following my procedure?			

Checklist 5: *What Does My Travel Companion Need to Do?*

A person who accompanies a health traveler gives a great gift. Here are some questions for potential companions to answer before they commit themselves to accompanying a health traveler abroad.

Travel companion's considerations	Yes	No	Not Sure
Am I sure I want to go? Am I sure I'm up to the task? (If you hesitate in answering either question, you may want to reconsider.)			
Am I willing and able to take responsibility for handling details, such as obtaining visas and passports?			
Do I feel comfortable acting as an advocate for the health traveler at times when he or she may need assistance?			
Have we agreed on the costs of the trip and on who is responsible for paying what?			
Do I feel sufficiently confident about handling experiences and challenges in a foreign country, such as getting through airports, arranging for taxis, or finding addresses?			
Do the health traveler and I communicate well enough to identify problems and solve them together amicably?			
Am I prepared to listen to and record doctor's instructions and provide reminders for the health traveler when needed?			
Can I help the health traveler stay in touch with family, friends, and healthcare providers back home?			
Have I allowed for "down time" and time for myself during the medical travel?			
Do I have the patience to help the health traveler through what might be a long and difficult recovery period, both abroad and back home?			

Part Two

Monterrey, Mexico: A Prime Destination for the Medical Traveler

---

Having read Part One, you now have a fair idea of what it takes to be a smart and informed health traveler. At this point, chances are you've already reached a decision about your course of treatment, and you may be seriously considering Monterrey as a destination for your medical care.

Part Two gives you an overview of Monterrey's developments and achievements as an international medical hub and provides in-depth information about the leading healthcare establishments, as well as health travel agents serving medical travelers to Monterrey.

Introduction

Each year, increasing numbers of global patients choose Monterrey as their medical travel destination. Why? Foremost these days, Monterrey is relatively safe compared to Mexico's border towns, where drug-related violence makes headlines on a regular basis. While Monterrey cannot claim to be untouched by conflict, medical travelers are safe when they entrust themselves to Monterrey's best hospitals, where transportation and accommodation services are provided to help ensure a safe journey.

Of equal importance is Monterrey's strong economy, with much of its affluence the direct consequence of the city's institutions of higher learning, combined with its status as headquarters for numerous multinational companies. This economic prosperity has encouraged the growth of private-sector hospitals that serve Monterrey's middle- and upper-class residents and—increasingly—a crowd of health travelers.

Modern Monterrey offers top-quality, yet inexpensive, treatment at American-accredited hospitals in the hands of well-trained doctors and surgeons. What's more, Monterrey lies within easy travel distance from the US, and it's a pleasant and engaging tourist destination.

Monterrey's Healthcare System

Monterrey is the capital of the northern Mexican state of Nuevo León. It's also home to four internationally significant universities: the Universidad Autónoma de Nuevo León (UANL), the third-largest university in Mexico; the Universidad de Monterrey (UDEM); the Universidad de Montemorelos (UM); and the Instituto Tecnológico y de Estudios Superiores de Monterrey (more commonly known as Tec de Monterrey, or TEC), widely considered to be Mexico's top university, either public or private.

Monterrey's healthcare, like the healthcare in all of Mexico, comprises three parallel and complementary systems:

1. Social security institutions (hospitals that are run by the government), which provide care for about 50 million Mexicans.
2. The Health Secretariat, which provides minimal services for the uninsured poor.
3. Private-sector hospitals, which provide services to those who can pay for them. These facilities serve approximately 3 million Mexicans, as well as thousands of health travelers annually.

Many private hospitals and dental clinics do not accept any form of foreign health insurance, but a few do. Cash or credit payment is required in advance by many as well, although there are exceptions there, too.

Several excellent medical centers operate in the smaller Mexican cities that are the favorite haunts of tourists. However, many private hospitals or clinics in rural areas are owned by groups of local physicians with varying levels of training. Rural facilities and technology are typically outdated but sufficient for managing minor illnesses. Patients with advanced care requirements are transferred to a tertiary medical center.

Monterrey's private hospitals provide some of the most advanced tertiary care in the world. Most of the doctors in these hospitals have excellent Mexican medical credentials, and many have trained abroad in Europe or the US. Among the shining stars of this sector is UANL, which runs Hospital Universitario Dr. José Eleuterio González. With a high-level shock-trauma unit and a specialized clinic for child cancer treatment, Universitario is recognized as the best public hospital in northeast Mexico, and its school of medicine is one of the best in the country. The other "biggest and best" are TEC, which runs Hospital San José Tec de Monterrey, and UDEM, which holds an alliance for medical and nursing education with the Christus Muguerza hospital group.

The presence of important research institutions means that Monterrey's hospitals are consistently on the cutting edge of new technologies and medical breakthroughs. In addition, Monterrey is home to four of Latin America's most prestigious schools of medicine (UANL, TEC, UDEM, and UM), which are answering the region's increasing demand for physicians. Many of the graduates from these schools complete internships at medical facilities in the US.

Why Monterrey Appeals to the Health Traveler

Warm weather, a beautiful setting, modern hospitals, and some of the best medical care in the world . . . what else could the health traveler ask for? Low prices! Monterrey has those, too. Depending on the medical procedure and the hospital chosen, prices in Monterrey can save the global patient 50–70 percent over the same treatment in the US and other countries. This excellent private healthcare system available at an affordable price means that medical tourism is encouraged and largely catered to. People come from as far away as Alaska and Hong Kong in search of bariatric, cosmetic, and cardiovascular procedures, as well as knee and hip replacements and more.

In general, the larger private healthcare facilities in Monterrey meet or exceed the best international standards of treatment and service. Such facilities offer the health traveler spotless hygiene, advanced technology, maximal efficiency, a complete choice of services and practitioners, little if any waiting time, high-quality care, and that all-important peace of mind that comes from knowing the doctor and hospital have passed rigorous scrutiny at the hands of accrediting agencies such as JCI. Furthermore, Mexico's last barrier to medical travel is quickly being dismantled: every year, more English-speaking physicians, nurses, translators, and case managers are available to serve the health traveler.

The pride of the medical community in Monterrey is threefold: state-of-the-art technology, the latest and most advanced procedures and techniques, and excellent training of medical personnel across all disciplines. All three of these assets have developed in tandem supported by the significant investment Monterrey has made in its infrastructure to facilitate the growth in its medical enterprises. In fact, Monterrey is Mexico's definition of opportunity. The city of 4 million *regios* (a nickname for Monterrey residents that means "people of the regal mountains") represents the future, as money has poured into northern Mexico from free trade and the opening of scores of assembly plants.

Other important factors for the medical traveler include ease of travel and comfort. Few destinations can rival Monterrey's convenient location. Direct flights are available from most US cities, and flights from New York take only 6 hours; from Los Angeles, they take 3. (Compare that to the 16–30 hours needed to reach Asia from the US.) In addition, Mexican hospitality is world-famous. International health travelers to Monterrey can expect to be welcomed warmly and treated kindly in this friendly city.

Specialties That Attract Medical Travelers to Monterrey

Monterrey offers the same specialties that attract medical travelers to other destinations. Such specialties are often elective surgeries that can be scheduled at the patient's convenience. They may also be procedures not typically covered by medical insurance policies. Monterrey's specialists are attracting bariatric, orthopedic, dental, and plastic surgery patients in large numbers. Monterrey offers cardiology, cardiovascular surgery, and cancer treatment, too. Infertile couples can find top-notch reproductive assistance and in vitro fertilization (IVF) in Monterrey at a fraction of the at-home price. Robotic-assisted surgery using the da Vinci system is also available at Monterrey's larger, high-tech hospitals, as are the latest technological innovations for ophthalmic surgery.

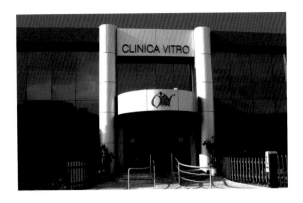
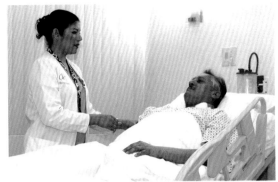
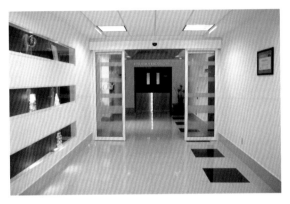
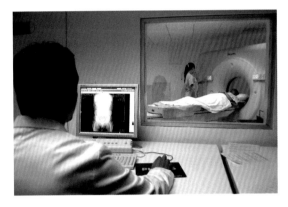
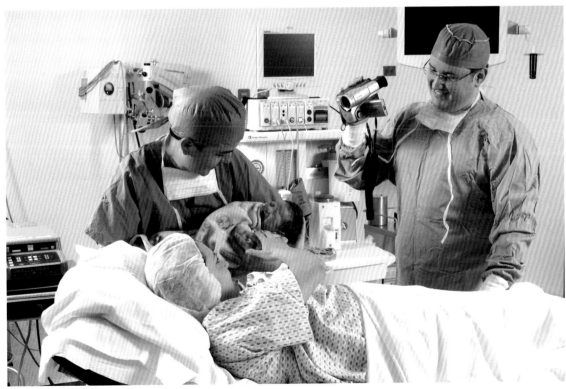

Clínica Vitro

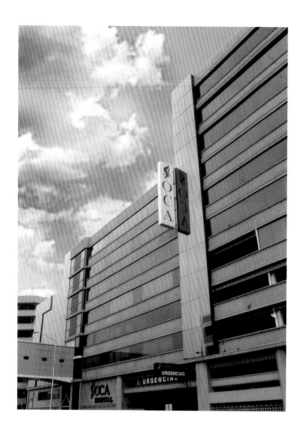

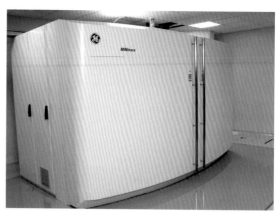

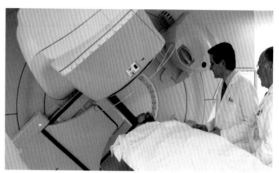

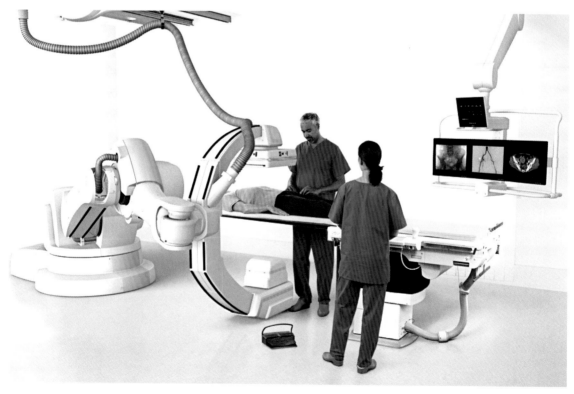

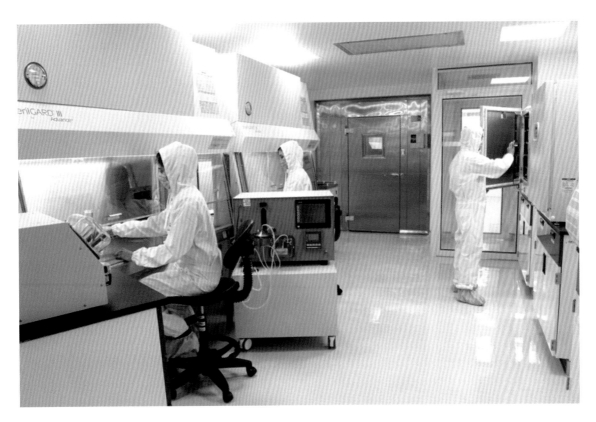

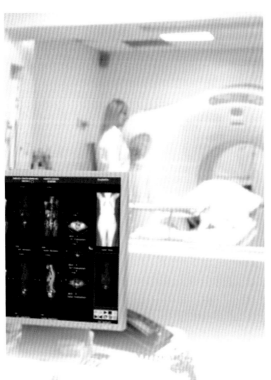

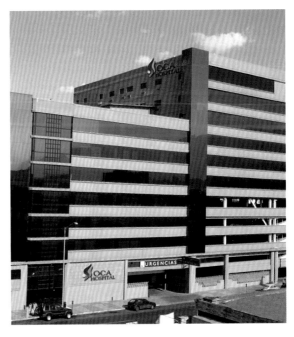

OCA Hospital

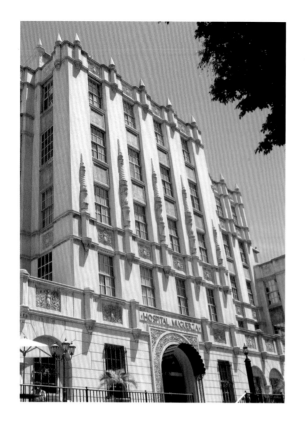
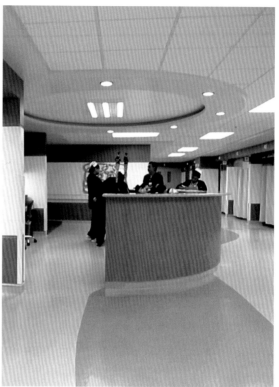
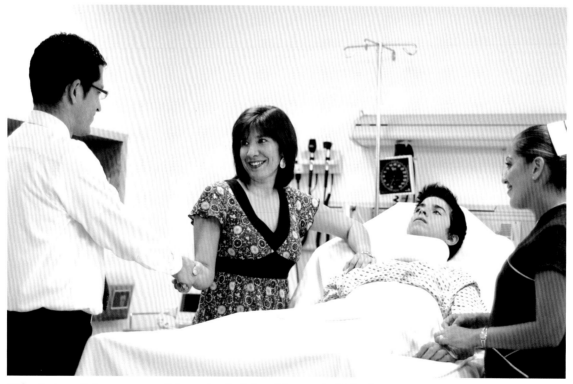

Christus Muguerza Hospital Alta Especialidad

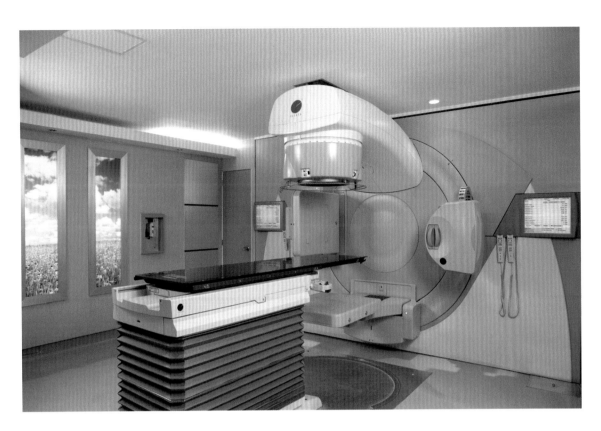

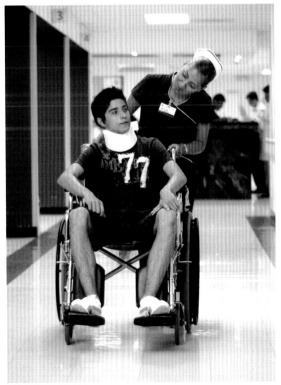

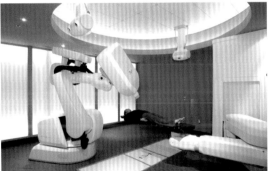

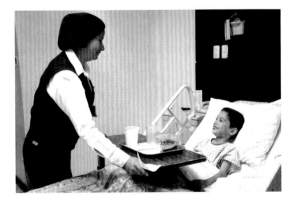

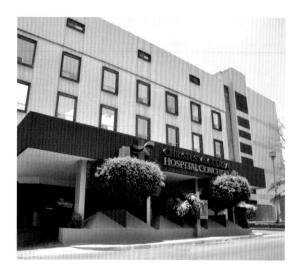

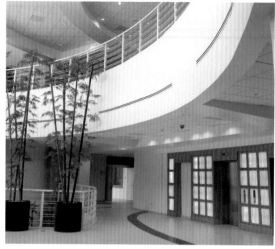

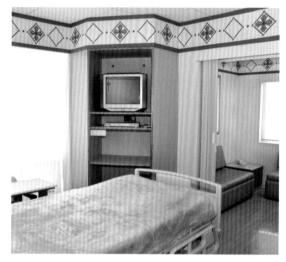

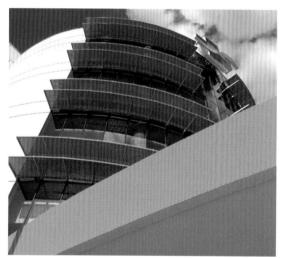

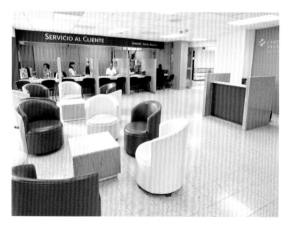

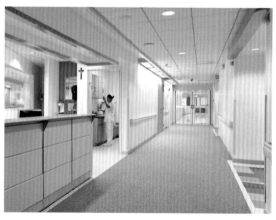

Christus Muguerza Hospital
Conchita, left column

Christus Muguerza Hospital Sur,
right column

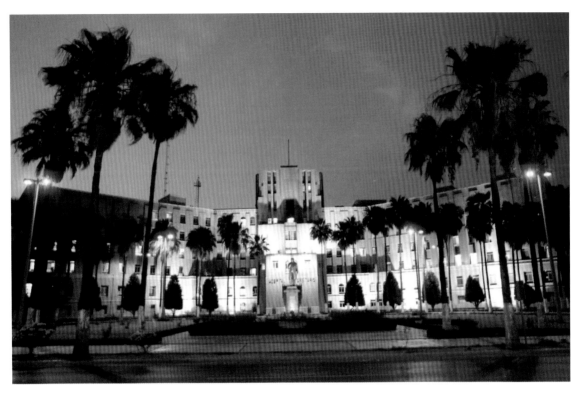

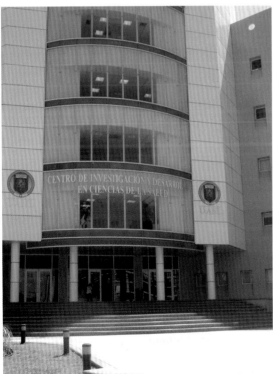

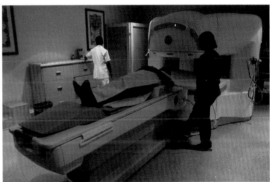

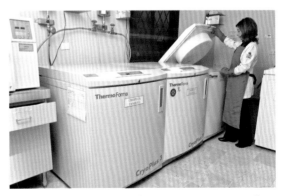

Hospital Universitario Dr. José Eleuterio González

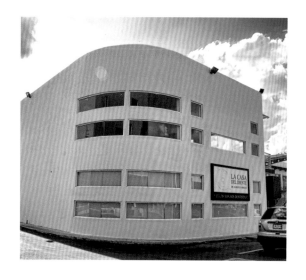
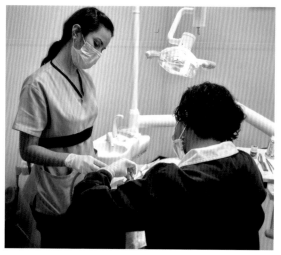
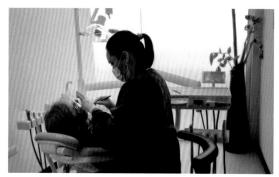
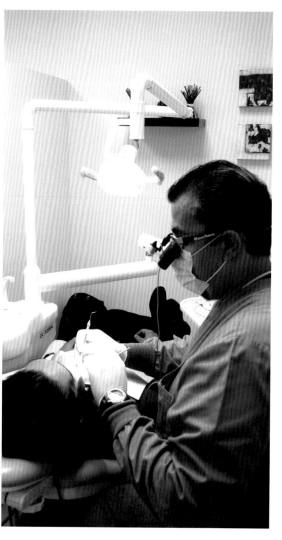
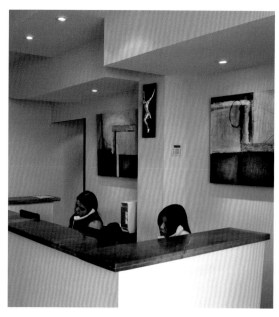

La Casa del Diente
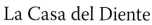

Featured Hospitals
in Monterrey, Mexico

Hospital Development in Monterrey

Altogether, ten hospitals or hospital groups and several dental clinics in Monterrey are targeting medical travelers or considering doing so, according to the Nuevo León Department of Tourism. Four hospitals hold current JCI accreditation: Christus Muguerza Hospital Alta Especialidad, Hospital CIMA Monterrey, OCA Hospital, and Hospital San José Tec de Monterrey. These and several others of Monterrey's finest healthcare facilities are described in this section.

Centro de Ginecología y Obstetricia de Monterrey (Ginequito)

Avenida Hidalgo Pte. #1842
Colonia Obispado
Monterrey, Nuevo León, MEXICO 64060
Tel: +52 81 8122.4700/4759
Email: comunica1@ginequito.com.mx
Web: ginequito.com.mx

Centro de Ginecología y Obstetricia de Monterrey, more widely and simply known as Ginequito, was established in 1976 and currently offers 63 patient beds. Thirty percent of its staff of 1,200 physicians and 199 nurses speak fluent English. The center performs approximately 1,420 outpatient procedures and 7,000 inpatient procedures annually, of which 150 are for international patients (about a third of them from the US). Ginequito provides specialty care in reproductive medicine, management of high-risk pregnancy, laparoscopic procedures, orthopedics, otolaryngology, plastic surgery, and weight loss surgery, among others.

Ginequito offers its patients five specialty clinics:

Profem Clinic The Profem Clinic provides comprehensive preventive care to women, men, teenagers, and children. Specific centers within the Profem Clinic offer advanced ultrasonography for detection of breast cancer, bone densitometry for detection of osteoporosis, pelvic echography, and more. Customized health screening programs provide complete medical evaluation and development of a preventive-health strategy. Packages are available, and testing is most often complete in one day.

Institute for the Study of Human Conception The Institute for the Study of Human Conception provides both counseling and treatment for infertility. Its Embryo and Gamete Laboratory maintains a high degree of quality control over all the center's services. Services include basic infertility exams, ovulation induction, artificial fertilization, and IVF. Female infertility is treated, as appropriate, with IVF, fresh or frozen embryo transfer, egg donation, egg freezing, embryo cultivation to blastocyst stage, and intrauterine insemination. Male infertility is treated, as recommended, via intracytoplasmic sperm injection, epididymis percutaneous aspiration, vasectomy reversal, sperm freezing, and semen banking.

Institute of Maternal-Fetal Medicine The Institute of Maternal-Fetal Medicine specializes in the management of high-risk pregnancies. Its pre-pregnancy services include ultrasound examinations of the breast, abdomen, reproductive organs, thyroid, and kidney, as well as family planning assistance and genetic counseling. Services for pregnant women include obstetric ultrasound, fetal echocardiography, and amniocentesis.

Center for Urology, Urodynamics, and Andrology The Center for Urology, Urodynamics, and Andrology specializes in urinary tract diseases. Treatment for prostatitis (prostate enlargement that causes difficulty in urinating) and prostate cancer is usually minimally invasive, such as state-of-the-art laparoscopy and cryoablation. The center's physicians also diagnose and treat lithiasis (calculi, or stones) in the urinary tract, often using a minimally invasive fragmentation procedure. Pediatric urologists specialize in the diagnosis and treatment of urological diseases in children. Other disorders handled at the center are interstitial cystitis, hyperactive bladder, urinary incontinence, enuresis, urinary infections, erectile dysfunction, premature ejaculation, and andropause.

Center for Obesity and Diabetes The newly opened Center for Obesity and Diabetes, also called REDUX, is the first of its kind in northern Mexico. It focuses on obesity treatment for adults and specially designed programs for children. Specialists in endocrinology are available for assessments and evaluation. The center also provides psychological and nutritional counseling for both medical and surgical patients. Surgical services include gastric band, gastric bypass, and intragastric balloon, as well as aesthetic-reconstructive plastic surgery for post-bariatric patients.

Ginequito's associated **Teaching and Research Center** offers subspecialty graduate degrees in fetal-maternal medicine, neonatology, and reproduction biology. Research focuses on women's reproductive health and neonatology. The center also provides continuing education opportunities for the hospital's medical staff.

Leading Specialties

- Bariatric surgery
- Diabetes prevention and management
- Gynecology (including gynecological laparoscopy)
- Neonatology
- Obstetrics (especially high-risk pregnancy)
- Orthopedics and traumatology
- Otolaryngology
- Pediatrics
- Plastic surgery
- Reproductive medicine and IVF
- Urology (adult and pediatric)

Selected Achievements and Awards

- Current: National Hospital Certification, awarded by the Department of Health, Mexico
- Current: Distintivo H certification, awarded by the National Secretary of Tourism for hygienic food handling
- 1987: Mexico's first birth using gamete intrafallopian transfer techniques
- 2007: Mexico's first birth from eggs preserved using the slow-freezing technique

Christus Muguerza Hospital Alta Especialidad

Avenida Hidalgo Pte. #2525
Colonia Obispado
Monterrey, Nuevo León, MEXICO 64060
Tel: +52 81 8399.3400; 1 866 558.6070, US and Canada toll-free
Email: internationalpatients@christusmuguerza.com.mx
Web: medicaltravel.com.mx, International Patient Services;
    christusmuguerza.com.mx, Spanish

Christus Muguerza Hospital (CMH) Alta Especialidad was established in 1935; it currently houses 200 patient beds. Many physicians and staff members speak English, and the dedicated, English-speaking team for international patients includes 32 internationally trained physicians. Together, the three CMH facilities in Monterrey employ more than 2,500 credentialed, specialized physicians and surgeons and more than 700 nurses.

CMH Alta Especialidad treats approximately 15,000 inpatients and 38,000 outpatients each year. The most frequently performed procedures are hip replacement, knee replacement, coronary bypass surgery, and spinal surgery. CMH Alta Especialidad specializes in cardiology and is Latin America's leading cardiac center. Additional top specialties include orthopedics, neurosurgery, oncology, and neonatology.

A number of important medical equipment providers work with the CMH group to drive technology-adoption programs for Latin America. These programs benefit patients through their doctors' access to the latest equipment available, including magnetic resonance imaging (MRI), a GE Innova 3100 15 hemodynamics system, and GE LightSpeed VCT series 64-slice computed tomography (CT) scanning for noninvasive cardiovascular imaging. An Elekta linear accelerator provides a treatment option for some cancer patients, and a Neuronavegador system is used in neurosurgery. With a total investment of US$6 million, CMH Alta Especialidad was the first hospital in Latin America to acquire the CyberKnife Robotic Radiosurgery System, which provides options for patients diagnosed with inoperable or surgically complex tumors and other patients looking for a noninvasive surgical treatment.

CMH Alta Especialidad's palliative care program has been designed and implemented to evaluate, treat, and follow up with holistic care for the physical, psychological, spiritual, and social needs of patients and their families, seeking to improve the patient's quality of life throughout treatment. The program involves nurses, nutritionists, psychologists, priests, pastoral agents, social workers, support groups, and many others.

Affiliated with US-based hospital system CHRISTUS Health, the Christus Muguerza group operates similarly to a US hospital network. CHRISTUS Health is ranked among the top ten largest Catholic health systems in the US and includes more than 40 hospitals and facilities in the US and Mexico. CMH is growing and expanding into rural areas. In eight years, two clinics in Monterrey were built and equipped, as well as a clinic in Zuazua, Nuevo León; a hospital in Tampamolón; and a clinic in Huichihuayán. Two new clinics are planned for Coahuila and Chihuahua.

Leading Specialties

- Cardiology and cardiovascular surgery
- Diabetes management
- Diagnostic imaging (including breast and cardiovascular)
- Neurology and neurosurgery
- Obstetrics and neonatology
- Oncology
- Orthopedics
- Physical and Neurological Rehabilitation Center (adult and pediatric)

Services Provided for International Patients

- Support from a dedicated international patient logistics coordinator
- Conference calls with physicians to discuss treatment options
- Detailed information about the procedure, physician, and price
- Assistance with flight schedules, travel arrangements, and hotel reservations

42   PATIENTS BEYOND BORDERS

- Free transportation to and from the airport; hotel-to-hospital transportation
- Concierge service, including hotel and sightseeing tour reservations
- Translation and interpretation
- Support from a nurse coordinator who manages all services, including communication with family, record-keeping and transmittal, and co-ordination of the discharge process

Selected Achievements and Awards

- Current: JCI accreditation
- Current: National Hospital Certification, awarded by the Department of Health, Mexico
- Current: Distintivo H certification, awarded by the National Secretary of Tourism for hygienic food handling
- Current: Distintivo M certification, awarded by the National Secretary of Tourism for quality management in cafeteria service
- Current: Clinical laboratory certification, awarded by the College of American Pathologists
- Current: Pathology/cytology laboratory certification, awarded by the College of American Pathologists
- Named one of the world's top ten best hospitals for medical tourists by the Medical Travel and Health Tourism Quality Alliance
- Named one of the international top five best hospitals for overseas healthcare by *Men's Health*
- Named a "Great Place to Work in Mexico" by the Great Place to Work Institute
- Named a "Super Company" by Grupo Expansión México

Feature Story

Paul H., Texas, United States
Christus Muguerza Hospital Alta Especialidad, Knee Surgery

Paul is a successful businessman—he runs a valet parking company—and an avid golfer; and both of these endeavors contributed to his knee problem, a meniscus tear that needed surgery. Paul had no insurance, so he decided to go south to Mexico where his surgery would be more affordable. Paul chose a JCI-accredited hospital in Monterrey for his surgery, and he is pleased with his choice. "It was the price, and also when I looked at the facility and at the service component. That's the problem with American hospitals: they have no service. They come across very sterile because of the way they have to handle things and be politically correct. The hospital I was at was very good. It seemed more sincere than the six major hospitals I've dealt with, doing different events as a valet parking contractor. It's different, their whole thing, the customer service."

Paul selected his surgeon based on his qualifications. "Qualifications were an important factor," Paul admits. "And then facilities, and how they handle things." Paul's anesthesiologist was a graduate of the University of Texas and did his residency at Southwest Medical. His surgeon, one of the top orthopedists in Mexico, was a graduate of Baylor (in the top 2 percent of his class), did his resi-

dency at St. Joseph's in Houston, and then went to UCLA. He also did a residency in San Antonio. Paul describes his surgeon: "Very matter-of-fact, and whatever I asked he understood, and he'd make sure I completely understood everything he told me. He's very sincere and loves what he does."

Paul made his own flight arrangements, and the hospital's international patient department took it from there, meeting Paul at the airport, taking him to his hotel, making calls for him, accompanying him through pre-op and the surgery itself, even calling Paul's business partner with updates on his status. The surgery went well, and he was walking around Monterrey the next day. And the savings were impressive. "It was six times less than what I would have paid in the US for a meniscus tear," Paul says. "There is no reason for a 40-minute meniscus-tear surgery to cost $30,000. I paid $5,100 for that, plus airfare and hotel. I think it's a wonderful way to have medical procedures done."

And six weeks later, he was able to return to his beloved game of golf. "I'd had a little bit of swelling but no pain during recovery, and you can't even see the scars from the scope. They gave me pain meds, but I never used them for the knee."

Paul was so impressed with his hospital in Monterrey that, when he decided he needed hand surgery, he didn't hesitate to book it there. This time, he was in considerable pain. "It got to the point where my finger was locking down like a money clip. So they went in and snipped it and relieved it. That second trip went as well as the first one. I flew in Sunday, had the surgery Monday, and flew out Tuesday. Very personal service."

Why should US visitors choose Monterrey? "Mexico has a geographical advantage over other destinations," says Paul. "Medical travel is limited in who's going to want to do it. It's not for every-body. People have to have an extremely open mind and attitude toward travel. I mean, I've talked to some people, even my doctor friends, and they're like, 'Oh, Mexico's really dangerous right now,' and I say, 'Well, so is Philadelphia and so is Dallas—it depends where you hang out.' I was escorted around, and they said, 'If you need anything, a car, whatever, just call us the night before.'"

Medical travel is right for him, Paul concludes. "All I did was talk to the international patient department, book my surgery, and book my own airfare. Simple. Two very short flights, and I was there." ■

Christus Muguerza Hospital Conchita

15 de Mayo #1822 Pte.
Colonia María Luisa
Monterrey, Nuevo León, MEXICO 64060
Tel: +1 52 81 8122.8122; 1 866 558.6070, US and Canada toll-free
Email: internationalpatients@christusmuguerza.com.mx
Web: medicaltravel.com.mx, International Patient Services;
    christusmuguerza.com.mx, Spanish

Christus Muguerza Hospital (CMH) Conchita was established in 1938 and joined the CMH group in 2003. It began as a hospital for women, but in recent years it has expanded to become a 100-bed general hospital that offers specialized care in pediatrics, neonatology, trauma, general surgery, plastic surgery, ear-nose-throat, and pediatric and adult intensive care. The hospital recently established a center of excellence in bariatric surgery. Gastric bypass and hysterectomy are the procedures most frequently performed.

CMH Conchita has 310 nurses and shares more than 2,500 specialized physicians across Christus Muguerza's three-hospital network in Monterrey. CMH Conchita serves nearly 18,000 outpatients (including emergency room visits and outpatient surgeries) and more than 6,500 inpatients per year. Of these inpatients, 70 are international bariatric patients from the US and Canada.

Leading Specialties
- Bariatric surgery
- General surgery
- Neonatology
- Obstetrics and gynecology
- Orthopedics
- Pediatrics

Services Provided for International Patients
- See "Christus Muguerza Hospital Alta Especialidad"

Selected Achievements and Awards

- Current: National Hospital Certification, awarded by the Department of Health, Mexico
- Current: Distintivo H certification, awarded by the National Secretary of Tourism for hygienic food handling
- Current: Distintivo M certification, awarded by the National Secretary of Tourism for quality management in cafeteria service

Christus Muguerza Hospital Sur

Carretera Nacional #6501
Colonia La Estanzuela
Monterrey, Nuevo León, MEXICO 64988
Tel: +52 81 8155.5000; 1 866 558.6070, US and Canada toll-free
Email: internationalpatients@christusmuguerza.com.mx
Web: medicaltravel.com.mx, International Patient Services;
    christusmuguerza.com.mx, Spanish

Christus Muguerza Hospital (CMH) Sur opened in 2006 with a novel building style emphasizing a bold, colorful interior and exterior. This bright, modern approach provides a refreshing contrast to more traditional, subdued hospital design. In 2009 CMH Sur opened its new neurophysiology department and a new-generation cardiac catheterization lab. The hospital boasts a tower with 120 consultation offices; medical areas for general surgery, trauma, cardiology, internal medicine, neurophysiology, endoscopy, pediatrics, and obstetrics; adult, pediatric, and neonatal intensive care units; and diagnostic support departments for imaging and hemodynamics.

Currently operating 51 beds, CMH Sur treats more than 18,000 outpatients (including emergency room visits and outpatient surgeries) and more than 3,500 inpatients annually, of whom about 80 are international patients, primarily from the US and Canada. The most frequently performed procedures are arthroscopy and bariatric surgery.

CMH Sur has 132 nurses and shares more than 2,500 specialized physicians across Christus Muguerza's three-hospital network in Monterrey. Members of the international patients' team speak English, as do many of the doctors and nurses.

Leading Specialties

- Addiction Treatment Center
- Bariatric surgery
- Dermatology Center
- General surgery
- Hemodialysis Center
- Obstetrics and gynecology
- Orthopedics
- Physical and Neurological Rehabilitation Center (adult and pediatric)
- Plastic surgery
- Wound Care Center and hyperbaric medicine

Services Provided for International Patients

- See "Christus Muguerza Hospital Alta Especialidad"

Selected Achievements and Awards

- Current: National Hospital Certification, awarded by Department of Health, Mexico
- Current: Distintivo H certification, awarded by the National Secretary of Tourism for hygienic food handling
- 2008: Named a "Great Place to Work in Mexico" by the Great Place to Work Institute
- 2009: Named a "Super Company" by Grupo Expansión México

Clínica Vitro

Escobedo #1405 Norte
Colonia Treviño
Monterrey, Nuevo León, MEXICO 64570
Tel: +52 81 8329.1800; +52 81 8329.1827
Email: sclientescvitro.com
Web: monterreyhealthcarecity.com/hospitals/clinica-vitro, English;
   clinicavitro.com, Spanish

Established in 1947, Clínica Vitro initially provided healthcare services for all Vitro employees and their families—Vitro is the leading glass manufacturer in Mexico and one of the largest in the world. In 2002 Clínica Vitro opened its doors to the general public. Now a tertiary-care hospital, Clínica Vitro offers a range of medical and surgical specialties and is affiliated with Memorial Hermann Hospital in Houston, Texas, as well as Universidad de Monterrey and Tec de Monterrey.

Clínica Vitro has 30 inpatient beds and a staff of 45 physicians and surgeons and 78 nurses who see about 77,550 outpatients and 2,760 inpatients every year. Clínica Vitro boasts a robust infrastructure, advanced imaging equipment, and a well-recognized clinical laboratory. Some of its physicians and staff speak English. The hospital's most frequently performed surgeries are bariatric, cosmetic, and orthopedic.

Leading Specialties
- Bariatric surgery
- Laparoscopic surgery
- Orthopedics (especially orthopedic surgery)
- Plastic and cosmetic surgery
- Urology

Selected Achievements and Awards

- Current: National Hospital Certification, awarded by the Department of Health, Mexico
- Current: Distintivo H certification, awarded by the National Secretary of Tourism for hygienic food handling
- Current: Clinical laboratory certification, awarded by Entidad Mexicana de Acreditación
- 2005: Nuevo León Award for Quality
- 2007: National Quality Award
- 2008: Iberoamericanco Award for Quality

Feature Story

Marty A., Washington, United States
Clínica Vitro, Bariatric Surgery

At age 64, Marty noticed she had become increasingly sedentary over the years. Climbing the stairs, taking a walk, or even plucking a weed in the garden was beyond her capabilities. Her diabetes was becoming insulin dependent, and a pain in her hip suggested that a joint replacement might be necessary soon. Her daughter had undergone gastric bypass surgery in the US a few years before, and Marty thought the procedure might help her, too. When she mentioned the possibility to her family doctor, the response was, "You're an excellent candidate; you're in good health, but you're obese." Marty knew she needed a major lifestyle change, but her insurance company would not cover the surgery, and she could not afford the US$60,000 cost estimate she was given at home.

Marty asked her daughter for help in researching surgical options in Mexico. "My grandfather was raised in Mexico, my parents wintered there, and we've been spending a couple weeks' vacation in the state of Jalisco for about 25 years," Marty explains. "When my father had a hip replacement at a private hospital in Guadalajara, his experience built my confidence in Mexico's medical system."

Marty and her daughter checked out support-group websites, did a Google search on hospitals offering gastric bypass, and evaluated the quality of hospitals, patients' reviews, and doctors' credentials. They found a bariatric surgeon at Clínica Vitro who had performed 4,000 gastric bypass operations over 15 years. The cost of the surgery, including hotel: US$10,000. "We figured those were pretty good statistics," Marty says.

Marty did not use a medical travel agency. She called the hospital directly, and the international relations department responded promptly, answering all her questions. Marty made a quick decision: "I spoke with them on October 1 and flew to Monterrey with my husband on October 11." An English-speaking employee of the hospital met the couple upon arrival and took Marty immediately to a laboratory for a blood draw. Next came an ultrasound to check for fat deposits around her liver. "We were then dropped off at a wonderful, comfortable hotel, and my surgery was confirmed for the following morning," Marty says.

Marty's operation went off without a hitch. "The hospital was very clean and had all the medical departments, so I knew they could take good care of me if I had any problems. The woman at the intake desk spoke English and was very professional. Upstairs, the anesthesiologist came in to meet me and answer my questions," Marty says. When she came out of surgery, she reunited with her husband, and the hospital staff made her comfortable in a private room. "The nurses were great. They didn't speak a lot of English, and I don't speak a lot of Spanish, but we did fine," she says. She subsequently spent six days recuperating in her hotel. "I had very little discomfort from the surgery," she says. "There was a sky-bridge over to a mall, so we walked and walked until my muscles were sore from the exercise. I was already losing 2 pounds a day."

Five months after her surgery, Marty lost 80 pounds and is enjoying excellent health. Her blood tests are normal, she has gone off the diabetic medication, and the pain in her hip has vanished. "I haven't needed a hip replacement after all; instead, I'm having physical therapy to strengthen my legs so they can do everything I expect of them," Marty says. She's dropped four dress sizes, and a friend has altered some of Marty's clothes for her—removing a whopping 18 inches! "It's a whole new life, and it's liberated me completely," Marty says. "In November, we visited our grandkids in California, and it was amazing, because we could walk to town and have a cup of coffee, and I could do it! I wouldn't even have tried it in the old days. I feel blessed."

Marty's finances also worked out well. She charged her procedure on her credit card, and she's already paid off the balance in full. Her family relationships are better, too. "My husband was so supportive throughout our trip, and he was great at helping me in and out of bed and checking tubes. It was good to have him right there. It actually made us closer, and as I keep losing weight, we're physically closer, too. He also lost about 25 pounds from the change in our lifestyle. It even saves us money, because we enjoy going out to eat, and now we can just agree on what we're sharing and split the meal."

Marty has lost so much weight that she may need plastic surgery to get rid of excess loose skin. If she does, and her insurance company won't pay, she plans to go back to Mexico, probably to the same hospital. Marty's advice to other medical travelers is to maintain a positive attitude. You have to say, "This is my mission and this is what I'm going to get done," just as Marty did. ∎

Hospital CIMA Monterrey

Frida Kahlo #180
Valle Oriente Garza García
Monterrey, Nuevo León, MEXICO 66260
Tel: +52 818 368.7777;
   Medical Value Travel Office: 1 866 540.3382, US toll-free
Email: intlpatientservices@cimamedicalvaluetravel.com
Web: cimamonterrey.com

The acronym CIMA stands for Centro Internacional de Medicina. Also a Spanish noun, *cima* means "peak" or "pinnacle," signifying not only the mountainous surroundings of the company's acute-care hospitals but also the high-quality healthcare they provide. CIMA Monterrey is part of the International Hospital Corporation (IHC) of Dallas, Texas, which has been in the international healthcare delivery industry for over a decade.

IHC owns and operates reputable healthcare facilities throughout Latin America. With a US-based management team and hospitals in Mexico, Costa Rica, and Brazil, IHC is uniquely positioned as the sole Pan-American leader in hospital-based healthcare. IHC runs 11 acute-care private hospitals: eight operating hospitals and three hospitals currently under development. Each is modeled after state-of-the-art facilities in the US, providing a full range of sophisticated surgical, emergency, and diagnostic services. The IHC-managed CIMA hospitals in Mexico and Costa Rica are JCI-accredited.

CIMA Monterrey was established in 1996. It currently has 70 beds (including intensive care and neonatal intensive care) with expansion capacity for 125 acute-care medical/surgical beds. The hospital is serviced by 2,706 credentialed physicians and surgeons and 180 nurses who treat about 27,000–30,000 outpatients and 4,500 inpatients per year. Physicians and staff members speak English; translation services are available for French, German, Italian, Japanese, and Korean.

Since its JCI accreditation in 2008, the hospital's international patient volume has grown by 70 percent annually, with approximately 90 percent of these patients coming from the US. CIMA Monterrey offers a complete array of diagnostic equipment, including multi-slice CT and open MRI systems capable of extra-fast scanning, decreasing the time patients are exposed to radiation and allowing physicians to view clearer images than ever before.

CIMA Monterrey was one of the first hospitals in Mexico to offer intensive care telemetry via the Internet. This enables a physician to see a patient's electrocardiogram and other vital signs from anywhere in the world in real time, in order to assess the patient's condition and quickly prescribe treatment within crucial minutes. CIMA Monterrey is affiliated with Southwestern Medical Center, University of Texas, Dallas, and the Mayo Clinic in Rochester, Minnesota; Jacksonville, Florida; and Phoenix, Arizona.

Leading Specialties

- Cardiology and cardiovascular surgery
- General surgery
- Gynecology
- Orthopedic surgery
- Otolaryngology (ENT)
- Plastic surgery
- Urology
- Weight loss surgery

Services Provided for International Patients

- Airport- and hospital-related transportation
- Hospital representative briefing of patient on medical agenda
- Concierge services on a fee-for-service basis
- International patient services center

Selected Achievements and Awards

- Current: JCI accreditation
- Current: National Hospital Certification, awarded by the Department of Health, Mexico

- Current: Distintivo H certification, awarded by the National Secretary of Tourism for hygienic food handling
- Current: Laboratory accreditation, awarded by PACAL, a program of external monthly evaluations of public and private labs nationwide for more than 20 years, to ensure and improve analytical quality

Feature Story

Al L., Georgia, United States
Hospital CIMA Monterrey and BridgeHealth, Bariatric Surgery

Al was having troubles with many facets of his health. He was extremely overweight, had diabetes and high blood pressure, and was tired and constantly falling asleep in the car or on the sofa. His doctor recommended a LAP-BAND, and Al thought that sounded fine . . . until he realized the cost: US$14,000 outpatient, US$17,000 inpatient, and none of it covered by his health insurance.

A woman in Al's office suggested a "medical vacation," something Al had never heard of. So he started doing research, contacting several groups in the US that assist people in medical travel. He also found some LAP-BAND discussion groups on Yahoo in which people who've had the surgery tell their stories and post their pictures. "I saw some interesting before-and-after pictures on there," Al says. The more Al studied the LAP-BAND option, the more right it seemed for him. "I didn't want any of the other bariatric options; I felt the LAP-BAND was the least intrusive," he explains.

Al had a number of concerns about having the procedure done abroad. For one thing, he needed to know who would fill his LAP-BAND back home. He felt sure no US doctor would touch him after he'd seen a doctor out of the country. But the medical travel company he selected reassured him on that point. It took the worry out of travel in several others ways, too, by taking care of Al's transportation and hotel arrangements. With Monterrey as his destination, he didn't need to be concerned about the Mexican border towns that made him uncomfortable.

"They sent me information on the doctor so I could evaluate him, and on the hospital, too," says Al. "It was an American-owned hospital, with American standards. The doctor does this procedure in Mexico and Texas, so on both sides of the border, which was reassuring. So I signed up with them. The whole thing ended up costing me $7,000 for travel and surgery in the hospital."

Al was a no-nonsense medical traveler. He wasn't interested in sightseeing: he just wanted to get the procedure done and go home to his wife. "They took me to the hotel [Tuesday] and said they'd pick me up early the next morning to do the pre-op blood work and everything," he explains. "They were there on time [Wednesday], took me to the hospital, I had the blood work, they took me back, and they picked me up again at 4:00 p.m. from the hotel and took me to the doctor's office. I met the doctor, and he told me everything that was going to happen.

"They picked me up the next morning [Thursday] around 5:30 a.m., took me to the hospital, and got me all checked in. The hospital is a beautiful, clean hospital. My room looked like an embassy suite, with a living area and whatnot. Another girl at the hospital was pretty much with me all the time after that. The anesthesiologist spoke good English and took me through the whole procedure. They rolled me in and did the operation, and a couple hours later I was out and back in my room. . . . Then I was back in the hotel on Friday. Saturday they took me to the airport and I was back home."

In spite of his prior misgivings about foreign travel, Al was impressed. "It was so professional, and it was so centered on me,

that I felt like I was being well taken care of at all times, and well looked after—better than I think I would feel in an American hospital. I mean, they treat you like you are someone very important who's having this done, and they're pleased to have your business," he says.

And the results were spectacular. "I've lost 72 pounds so far. I'm feeling a world of difference. I can bend over and tie my shoes . . . I mean, not having to get down on one knee to tie my shoe and not breathing hard to do it. As a result of this surgery, I've eliminated all my diabetes medicine, and I've cut my blood pressure medicine in half, and I'm not even sure I need it, or even sure I need the Lipitor that I take. I took Prevacid for reflux for 15 years, and I don't take that anymore either. I am 65 and I feel like I'm 50."

He's feeling, in fact, like a different person. "The side effect that I was having with the diabetes medicine was sporadic diarrhea, so every place I went I had to check for the bathroom, and it was a real drag. So it's like a whole different life. I couldn't watch TV before without falling asleep. Now I have to take something at night to go to sleep, because of my energy level! And there's been no pain in my recovery." ■

OCA Hospital

Pino Suaréz #645 Norte
Colonia Centro
Monterrey, Nuevo León, MEXICO 64000
Tel: +52 81 8262.0000
Email: informacion@ocahospital.com
Web: monterreyhealthcarecity.com/hospitals/hospital-oca, English;
   ocahospital.com, Spanish

OCA stands for Organización Clínica América (Organizational Clinic of America). Hospital OCA was established in 1973 with only 30 beds and a 100-person staff. Today it has grown into a tertiary-care hospital with nearly 300 beds, 25 operating rooms, and 24 emergency beds attended by 2,000 physicians and surgeons, 500 nurses, and 150 additional staff. The hospital treats about 100,000 outpatients and 30,000 inpatients every year, of whom 300 are international patients (95 percent from the US and Canada). The hospital's most frequently performed procedures are gallbladder removal, appendectomy, and radiotherapy. Some of the physicians and staff speak English.

Known for exceptional medical technology, OCA's nuclear medicine department boasts two of the most advanced gamma cameras: the Infinia and the Xeleris II with CT image processing. Unlike traditional anatomical imaging, a gamma camera can show physiological functions, which can help to identify disease processes by organ system. Other equipment includes a Philips iU22 ultrasound, an iE33 ultrasound, Angiotac 1.5-Tesla Intera and Philips Achieva 3.0T magnetic resonance imaging (MRI) scanners, and numerous digital x-ray machines. These innovations support diagnosis and treatment of infectious diseases, cancer, heart and cardiovascular disorders, neurological abnormalities, and dysfunctions of the endocrine system. OCA was the first hospital in Mexico to obtain a positron emission tomography (PET)–CT scanner with a cyclotron. Philips Healthcare, GE Healthcare, and Miltenyi Biotech have recognized OCA as a Center of Technological Excellence.

OCA was the first North American hospital to conduct laser diode spinal surgery, the first Latin American center to perform single-session radiosurgery, and the only private hospital to achieve genetic coding of the H1N1 virus. OCA's affiliated **Monterrey International Research Center** (MIRC) focuses on development of new cancer therapies.

Leading Specialties

- Cardiology
- General surgery
- Neurology and neurosurgery
- Oncology
- Orthopedics

Services Provided for International Patients

- Transportation to and from the airport
- Hotel shuttle
- Translation

Selected Achievements and Awards

- Current: JCI accreditation
- Current: National Hospital Certification, awarded by the Department of Health, Mexico
- Current: Distintivo H certification, awarded by the National Secretary of Tourism for hygienic food handling
- 2007: Nuevo León Award for Quality
- 2008: Named as a Technological Reference Center for Latin America by Philips Healthcare
- Mexico's first PET-CT scanner with cyclotron
- Northern Mexico's first clinical research center
- Mexico's first intracoronary stem cell implant in an infarcted heart for tissue regeneration, with excellent results

- Latin America's first single-session radiosurgery
- Northern Mexico's first pediatric liver transplant
- North America's first spinal diode laser surgery

Hospital San José Tec de Monterrey

Avenida Ignacio Morones Prieto #3000 Pte.
Colonia Los Doctores
Monterrey, Nuevo León, MEXICO 64710
Tel: +52 81 8347.1010; +52 81 8389.8390; 1 866 475.6334, US and Canada
  toll-free
Email: cfuentes@hsj.com.mx; international@hsj.com.mx
Web: international.hsj.com.mx

Hospital San José Tec de Monterrey, established in 1969, has since grown into one of Latin America's finest medical facilities. The hospital now has 200 beds (including 11 master suites and 96 junior suites in the tower), 38 intensive care beds, and 21 emergency beds. More than 1,500 affiliated physicians and about 500 nurses treat approximately 15,000 inpatients and 92,000 outpatients at San José Tec annually, including 1,400 international patients (800 from the US and Canada). Physicians and staff members speak English, French, and Spanish. More than 90 percent of the doctors have worked at US or European hospitals. The hospital's five centers of excellence are cardiology, oncology, neuroscience, organ transplant, and liver disease. The most frequently performed procedures are general surgeries, gastric bypass (Roux-en-Y), LAP-BAND, breast imaging, robotic-assisted surgery, prostate surgery, radiotherapy, and chemotherapy.

San José Tec's specialized surgical unit has 11 "intelligent operating rooms" designed for the most complex medical procedures. Its state-of-the-art emergency room coordinates with a medical transport network (hospital, land ambulance, air ambulance) that covers the entire continent. Modern medical equipment at San José Tec includes the ophthalmologic surgery unit's cutting-edge microscope and sophisticated excimer laser, YAG laser, and Nd Zeiss argon laser systems. Zeiss OPMI NC-4 microscope equipment is used for neurosurgery and spinal cord surgery. The hospital also owns and operates a da Vinci robotic-assisted surgery system. A linear accelerator enables conventional radiation therapy, intensity-modulated radiotherapy, and stereotactic radiosurgery. The cardiac catheterization laboratories are equipped with digital technology to perform endovascular and hemodynamic therapy. San José Tec obtains images using PET, CT, and 2-Tesla MRI scanning as required. Digital angiography aids in the diagnosis and surgical treatment of heart, brain, and peripheral arteries.

San José Tec enjoys a cardiology partnership with the Methodist Hospital DeBakey Heart and Vascular Center in Houston, Texas. The school of medicine also has reciprocal training programs with Johns Hopkins Medicine in Baltimore, Maryland; and Baylor College of Medicine in Houston, Texas. Through its medical school, its **Center for Biotechnology**, and its **Center for Innovation and Technology Transfer**, San José Tec educates healthcare professionals and develops new models for clinical care and research. The hospital's **Zambrano Hellion Medical Center** opened in 2010, housing institutes for oncology, cardiology, and vascular medicine. San José Tec is currently developing the **Salvador Sada Gomez Center for Geriatrics and Alzheimer's Disease**, a facility combining research, teaching, and patient care.

Leading Specialties

- Cardiology and vascular medicine
- General, laparoscopic, and robotic-assisted surgery
- Hepatology (liver)
- Neurology and neurosurgery
- Oncology, including chemotherapy and radiotherapy
- Organ transplantation

Services Provided for International Patients

- Dedicated customer service office for international patients
- Detailed information about medical treatments, services, and payment options
- Assistance with flight schedules, travel arrangements, and hotel reservations
- Free transportation to and from the airport and between the hotel and hospital
- Administrative support, including pre-admission, admission, and discharge
- Translation and interpretation assistance

Selected Achievements and Awards

- Current: National Hospital Certification, awarded by the Department of Health, Mexico
- Current: Distintivo H certification, awarded by the National Secretary of Tourism for hygienic food handling
- Current: Multi-Organ Transplant Center certification, awarded by the Secretary of Health for all types of organ transplants, the only center of its kind in Mexico
- Current: Bone Marrow Transplant certification, awarded by the National Marrow Donors Program
- 2010: Multi-Organ Transplant Center's first "split" liver transplant, simultaneously benefiting a pediatric patient at the Instituto Mexicano del Seguro Social and an adult patient at San José Tec
- Recognized by Siemens as a Center of Excellence in Mexico

Feature Story

Brandy K., Indiana, United States
Hospital San José Tec de Monterrey, Bariatric Surgery

Brandy is a financial aid officer at her local community college; she lives with her twin 12-year-old sons and her disabled mother.

"My problem was that I was morbidly obese. At 5'3" I weighed 355 pounds. I've never been bedridden due to my weight, but walking was exhausting and painful. I couldn't play with my sons. I didn't have the energy to go to events with them. I was never enthusiastic about the prospect of being seen by a lot of people. We never went on vacations that would require me to fit into a narrow seat. I avoided movie theaters and restaurants with booths. It restricted what I felt I could do with my sons, so we stayed home entirely too often."

Although she had medical insurance through her job, two applications and two refusals made it clear that Brandy's insurance would not pay for bariatric surgery. A friend said to her, jokingly, "Why not go to Mexico?"

Why not, indeed? thought Brandy. Her first move was to Google the terms "bariatric surgery Mexico." Through that, she found links to several medical travel facilitators in Monterrey. She identified an agency that had an informative and professional website and offered facilitation for more than just bariatric surgery. "This was something I was looking for," Brandy says. "Their scope is comprehensive, rather than focusing on a single type of surgery. In my mind, this meant they were far less likely to be a front for a single surgeon who simply funnels people into his own practice."

Brandy talked to friends, family, and her own doctor about her choices and did comprehensive research before making a commitment. Her medical travel agent communicated with her through both email and phone calls. "[My agency] understood that I was only willing to have surgery done in a hospital," she says. "They collected my information and sent me a packet that included the bios of surgeons who fit my needs and specifications. They acted as a liaison between me and my chosen surgeon." Brandy secured her surgeon's résumé and took it with her when she went to see her personal physician at home. Her plan was nearly complete.

Her medical travel agency would have booked a hotel for her, but that detail was handled by a friend. A representative of Brandy's agency met Brandy's plane at the airport and took her to her hotel. He explained to Brandy what she could expect and stayed with her as both support and interpreter through all her pre-surgical lab tests. "I think the most touching and surprising thing he did was to sit next to me all the way up until I was wheeled into the operating room," Brandy says. "It was incredibly comforting to have him there to talk to. I'll never forget it. Surgery is scary no matter where you have it done. He made me feel like I was at home and in the best of hands."

Brandy was delighted with both her hospital and her surgeon in Monterrey. "If I could go to him for every surgery, every medical question, every ache or pain, I would!" Brandy exclaims. "He answered every email I sent to him before my surgery (and believe me, there were dozens). He called me on the phone. He came to see me every single day that I was in Mexico. He came to my hospital room. He came to my hotel room. He answered his cell phone no matter where he was or what time of day it was. Still to this day, he emails me to check up on me. It has been ten months since I last saw him. He's my angel."

And the hospital receives its share of praise as well: "It's a beautiful facility. It isn't just clean; it's spotless. There's an art gallery in the lobby. There's art hanging in the hallways. Gorgeous art. I didn't meet a single unfriendly member of the staff. I never had a language barrier. I saw touch-screen computer technology that I'd never seen at home. I saw waiting rooms that are simply unparalleled in any hospital I've ever been in before. My hos-

pital room was very pretty and had an amazing view of the mountains. The staff was so quick to respond to any need. It was fantastic."

Brandy's surgery went smoothly. "I didn't have excessive pain," she reports. "By that, I mean that the pain I experienced was not unexpected for my procedure. [My doctor] made sure I had access to good pain medicine to manage my discomfort. As a matter of fact, just days after surgery, I was able to hike up a gently sloping mountain to see a waterfall. After that, my friends and I walked through at least a couple of miles of roadside shopping booths. It was hot and I was tired, but I didn't hurt."

And she's had no complications or problems with followup care. "I had the best medical attention I've ever had in my life while I was in Mexico," she says. And her medical travel experience has given her new confidence. "I know now that I can get into the country without a problem, I can get out of the country without a problem, I can navigate the city and the language barriers without a problem, and I can be seen by excellent physicians without a problem."

While Brandy does consider herself fortunate, she does not attribute the success of her experience to luck. She credits her doctor, her hospital, and her health travel agent for the excellence of the healthcare services they provide. ∎

Hospital Universitario Dr. José Eleuterio González

Avenida Madero y Gonzalitos S/N
Colonia Mitras Centro
Monterrey, Nuevo León, MEXICO 64460
Tel: +52 81 8369.1111
Email: eperez@hospitaluniversitario.org
Web: www.medicina.uanl.mx

Hospital Universitario Dr. José Eleuterio González is the clinical adjunct to Universidad Autónoma de Nuevo León (UANL). Named in honor of UANL's founder, Universitario is a multidisciplinary medical institution offering 53 departments and the latest medical technology. With ten buildings dedicated to patient care, the hospital has 425 beds and is staffed by 249 professors, 400 medical residents, and 692 nurses. Seventy percent of the staff speak English.

Universitario handles all levels of medical care and treats more than 19,000 inpatients and 250,000 outpatients each year, with 40,000 emergency room visits. It is the largest emergency and specialization hospital in northeast Mexico. Its clinics and departments include general surgery, genetics and birth defects, gynecology and obstetrics, sports medicine, family medicine, internal medicine, clinical pathology, pediatrics, and radiology and imaging. Additional areas of specialty include psychiatry, orthopedics, dermatology, urology, endocrinology, cardiology, neurology, otorhinolaryngology, and neurosurgery.

Leading Specialties

- Oncology and hematology
- Ophthalmology
- Organ transplantation and bone marrow bank
- Radiology and imaging
- Reproductive medicine

Selected Achievements and Awards

- Current: National Hospital Certification, awarded by the Department of Health, Mexico
- Certification by the Mexican Council for Accreditation of Medical Education
- Accreditation of all undergraduate and graduate programs

La Casa del Diente

Avenida Revolución #3780 L-1
Colonia Torremolinos
Monterrey, Nuevo León, MEXICO 64850
Tel: +52 81 8348.5500, +52 81 8354.1010
Email: cvillarreal.lcdd@gmail.com
Web: lacasadeldiente.com

La Casa del Diente comprises six dental clinics in the Monterrey metropolitan area. Established in 1984, "the Home of Teeth" has 110 certified dentists and dental surgeons. They see approximately 24,000 new patients every year, of whom 130 are international (110 from the US and Canada). The most frequently performed procedures at La Casa del Diente include cosmetic treatments, dental implants, and porcelain veneers. A notable innovation in these clinics is the "Wand" computer-controlled technology for local anesthesia, eliminating the need for syringes. Most of the dentists and staff members speak English. Special package plans for medical travelers include treatment, accommodations, transfers, and the services of a bilingual assistant.

Leading Specialties

- Cosmetic dentistry
- Endodontics
- Implants
- Orthodontics
- Periodontics
- Porcelain veneers
- Reconstruction
- Whitening

Health Travel Agents Serving Monterrey, Mexico

MedRetreat

2042 Laurel Valley Drive
Vernon Hills, IL 60061
Tel: +1 443 451.9996; 1 877 876.3373, US toll-free
Email: customerservice@medretreat.com
Web: medretreat.com

In operation since 2003, MedRetreat is one of the better-established US-based health travel agencies, sending patients to Argentina, Brazil, Costa Rica, El Salvador, India, Malaysia, Mexico, South Africa, and Thailand. Members receive personalized service through a boutique-style program designed to meet their specific needs. This process includes acquiring hospital information, physicians' credentials, and doctors' consultations; collecting and disseminating medical records; completing price quotations; and arranging procedures, passport and visa acquisition, air travel, travel insurance, financing, destination ground transportation, post-operative hotel booking, and more. MedRetreat provides 24-hour access to a US program manager, concierge services in the treatment destination, communications while abroad, and assistance once back home. MedRetreat also offers assistance in locating a finance company and an unconditional money-back guarantee.

Satori World Medical

591 Camino de La Reina, #407
San Diego, CA 92108
Tel: +1 619 704.2000, 1 800 613.9686, US toll-free
Email: info@satoriworldmedical.com
Web: satoriworldmedical.com

Satori World Medical started operating in 2007, and its growing network includes hospitals in Costa Rica, India, Mexico, the Philippines, Singapore, and Thailand. Satori's staff members speak English, Farsi, Japanese, and Spanish. The agency's patient advocates are nurses who coordinate all inquiries, from discussing procedures with the patient and facilitating medical records–transfer to scheduling followup care and educating companions on their responsibilities. The agency's travel-care coordinators schedule procedure dates with the hospital, make airline and hotel reservations, coordinate ground transportation, and provide 24-hour customer service. Satori's clients include self-funded employers, health plans, unions, trusts, municipalities, third-party administrators, benefit brokers, and consultants. Package pricing includes all procedure, hospital, and physician fees; round-trip airfare for the patient and a companion; a two-week hotel stay; and a personal accident insurance policy.

WorldMed Assist

1230 Mountain Side Court
Concord, CA 94521
Tel: 1 866 999.3848, US toll-free
Email: info@worldmedassist.com
Web: worldmedassist.com

Since opening in 2006, WorldMed Assist has established partnerships with several hospitals and has become the medical logistics provider for clients of Swiss Re's Commercial Insurance. It serves about 40 patients each month—nearly all of them from the US and Canada—with arrangements for medical care in Belgium, India, and Mexico. The agency aims to provide the highest possible level of customer service, with case management handled by registered nurses, not salespeople. Staff members speak English and Spanish. WorldMed advertises highly competitive rates with no markups on surgeries, and it conducts negotiations on the client's behalf with its ongoing partners. The agency and its clients have been featured on BBC, ABC News, Fox News, and NPR's *All Things Considered*.

Part Three

Traveling in Monterrey, Mexico

International travel can be a life-changing experience, and medical travelers can bring back more from their trip than improved health: they can return with an appreciation for a landscape, a culture, and a way of life very different from their own.

In Monterrey, international patients and their companions can find many different ways to enjoy this historic "City of the Mountains." From the breathtaking pink marble Palacio de Gobierno to the Museo del Vidrio (Glass Museum) to the IMAX dome at the Planctario Alfa, there is plenty to see and do! Shoppers will find the best in handmade leather goods, and diners can take their pick among a host of fine restaurants. The mountains surrounding Monterrey attract hikers, rock climbers, spelunkers, and bikers. Or maybe, while you are recovering, you'd just like to drink in the scenery from your hotel balcony!

Part Three provides important details to help you plan your medical journey to Monterrey, along with some ideas for enjoying the country's unique sights and experiences while you're there.

Monterrey, Mexico in Brief

Monterrey is located in Mexico's northeast desert area, at the edge of the Sierra Madre Oriental mountain range. It is Mexico's third-largest city, sometimes called the Sultan of the North or the City of the Mountains.

Monterrey has played host to a number of world-class events. In 2002 Monterrey welcomed the United Nations Conference on Financing for Development; the participation of more than 50 heads of state, as well as other ministers and senior delegates from more than 150 countries, resulted in the adoption of the Monterrey Consensus, a reference point for international development and cooperation. In 2004 the Organization of American States' Special Summit of the Americas in Monterrey was attended by almost all the presidents of the Americas. In 2007 Monterrey held the Universal Forum of Cultures with 4 million visitors.

A Brief History

Before European settlers arrived in what would become Nuevo León, nomadic tribes left cave paintings and petroglyphs in the area; but Monterrey's recorded history officially begins in 1596. That's when Spaniard

Diego de Montemayor led a small group of families to where the Museo de Historia Mexicana (Museum of Mexican History) now stands. There they officially founded the Ciudad Metropolitana de Nuestra Señora de Monterrey, and Montemayor served as governor of the region for more than 20 years. He probably chose Monterrey's site because of the presence of a natural fountain that could supply the new settlement with clean water, a priceless commodity in an arid region.

Spanish rule lasted until the Mexican War of Independence, and during this time Monterrey established itself as a trade center in partnership with San Antonio, Texas, which in turn served as the gateway north to British and French colonies. The War of Independence, lasting from 1810 to 1821, devastated the country. Despite the conflict, Monterrey was poised to become a key economic center for Mexico. It survived the civil war as well as two subsequent invasions from the North, including the 1846 Battle of Monterrey, in which hand-to-hand battles were fought in the city itself.

General Bernardo Reyes became provisional governor after the invasions; he brought stability to the region through an autocratic rule, encouraging economic development and industrialization. During his tenure, the railway system extended Monterrey, opening up many new trade possibilities. During this period, José Eleuterio González founded the Hospital Civil, today one of the best public hospitals in northeast Mexico and serving a prominent school of medicine in Nuevo León.

Geography

The Monterrey basin area and most of the surrounding mountains are brown and rocky, dotted with shrubs that are brown most of the year, turning green only after periods of hard rainfall. Myriad canyons, roads, and trails cross both deserts and forests in the mountains surrounding Monterrey. You probably won't see the Río Santa Catarina, which bisects Monterrey—the river is usually dry on the surface, but it has a significant underground flow.

Monterrey lies north of the foothills of the Sierra Madre Oriental. A small hill, the Cerro del Topo, and the even smaller Topo Chico are located in the suburbs of San Nicolás de los Garza and Escobedo. West of the city rises the Cerro de las Mitras (Mountain of the Miters), named for its silhouette—it looks a little like a row of bishops. At 6,800 feet (2,073 meters), it's nearly a mile higher than the city and its surroundings.

The Cerro de la Silla (Saddle Mountain) dominates the view southeast of the city; it is the most striking and recognized Monterrey landmark and a popular hiking destination. Its elevation of 5,971 feet (1,820 meters) raises it some 4,200 feet (1,280 meters) above the city.

To the south, the imposing Sierra Madre Oriental range reaches heights of up to 12,300 feet (3,750 meters) above sea level—an impressive 2 miles (3,220 meters) above the Monterrey metropolis and surrounding area. These mountains are part of the Parque Nacional Cumbres de Monterrey, a national park.

Weather and Climate

Monterrey's climate is arid, with rainfall scarce: the annual rainfall averages only about 23 inches (less than 60 centimeters), most of which falls between June and October. September receives the most rainfall, an average of just over 5 inches (12 centimeters) of rain (nearly three times the average of the other months).

Temperatures are extreme: August's thermometer readings can climb into the high nineties and low hundreds (Fahrenheit). December's temperatures, on the other hand, can dip down as far as freezing, though the average is closer to the mid-forties.

During the rainy season, rain tends to fall in late afternoons, in short, intense storms that may last from 5 to 30 minutes. Watch out for street flooding! Drainage is still not adequate for the city, and floods can easily reach depths of 2 feet (more than half a meter). Be careful and avoid underpasses and low-lying areas when it's been raining hard.

Festivals

Public celebrations are ingrained in Latin American culture, and Monterrey's calendar is filled with events that tempt residents and visitors alike. Popular festivals include the Festival Internacional de Títeres (International Puppet Festival) in July, the Festival Internacional de Cine de Monterrey (Monterrey International Film Festival) in August, and a trade fair called Expo Monterrey each September.

A City of Intellect

Monterrey's population of over 4 million people is the most educated in Mexico. On a per capita basis, more colleges, universities, and institutes of technology operate in Monterrey than in any other city in Mexico. In 2005 the city had 72 public libraries!

Monterrey is the headquarters of the Instituto Tecnológico y de Estudios Superiores de Monterrey (Monterrey Institute of Technology and Higher Studies), one of the most important private universities in Mexico and the country's equivalent of the Massachusetts Institute of Technology. The Universidad Autónoma de Nuevo León (Autonomous University of Nuevo León) is the third-largest Mexican university, with a system that includes 26 colleges, 22 graduate divisions, 24 high schools, a center of bilingual education, and three technical high schools. It boasts one of the most advanced medical schools in Latin America.

In 1969 the Universidad Regiomontana—a private university offering high school, undergraduate, and graduate programs—was founded with the help and financial support of local leading multinational corporations, including CEMEX, ALFA, FEMSA, Gamesa, Protexa, and Cydsa. It has reciprocal agreements with 200 international universities and is a member of the Global Alliance for Transnational Education and the Federación de Instituciones Mexicanas Particulares de Educación Superior. Its urban location attracts many working professionals as mature students who bring worldly experience and knowledge to the campus.

The Universidad de Monterrey was founded by the religious congregations of the Sisters of Immaculate Mary of Guadalupe, the nuns of the Sacred Heart, and the Marist and La Salle Brothers; it's further supported by an association of Catholic citizens. It was accredited in 2001 by the Southern Association of Colleges and Schools to deliver bachelor's and master's-level educational programs.

Language and Culture

The official and prevailing language of Monterrey is Spanish, spoken by the majority of the population. Some English is spoken, particularly by those involved in the healthcare delivery system. Mexican culture in general is a rich, complex blend of Native American, Spanish, and American traditions. In much of the country, rural areas are populated by descendants of the Maya, Aztec, and Toltec tribes, and by Spanish and mestizo farmers and laborers; each of these heritages has enriched the regional culture. In Monterrey itself, however, the primary influence is Spanish.

Monterrey boasts some of Mexico's finest museums and galleries. Many contemporary artists are producing identifiably Mexican work that blends Spanish, Native American, and modern European styles. The Mexican literary community has contributed such noted twentieth-century writers as novelists Mariano Azuela, Martín Luis Guzmán, Andrés Henestrosa, Agustín Yáñez, and Carlos Fuentes; playwrights Víctor Barroso and Rodolfo Usigli; and poets and essayists Alfonso Reyes and Octavio Paz. (Paz won the Nobel Prize in Literature in 1990.)

Mexican musicians, notably the composer and conductor Carlos Chávez, have received critical acclaim throughout the world. The Orquesta Sinfónica Nacional (National Symphony Orchestra) was founded in 1928 by Chávez, and the Ballet Folklórico in 1952 by the choreographer Amalia Hernández. Distinctive folk songs and dances are accompanied by several kinds of guitar-based ensembles. The ubiquitous *mariachi*, or popular strolling bands, are typically composed of two violins, two five-string guitars, a *guitarrón* (large bass guitar), and a pair of trumpets.

Business Development

In 1999 Monterrey was identified by *Fortune* magazine as the best city in Latin America in which to do business. More than 13,000 companies in Monterrey produce nearly 10 percent of Mexico's manufactured products and 30 percent of the country's manufactured exports. Monterrey accounts for about 95 percent of the gross domestic product (GDP) of the state of Nuevo Léon and 8.6 percent of Mexico's total GDP. Excluding telecommunications and oil monopolies, Monterrey controls more than half of Mexico's total industrial assets.

Imports are very high due to the area's strong manufacturing base and geographical proximity to the US. Imports are estimated at US$20 billion in goods alone, approximately 74 percent of US origin. Monterrey figures prominently in sectors such as steel, cement, glass, auto parts, and brewing. The city has become an important industrial and business center, serving as operations host for an array of Mexican companies that includes PEMEX, Lanix Electronics, CEMEX, Vitro, Zonda Telecom, Mercedes-Benz-Valdez, OXXO, Mastretta, BMW de México, and Alestra Telecom. Monterrey is also home to such international companies as Sony, Toshiba, Whirlpool, Samsung, Toyota, Ericsson, Nokia, Dell, Boeing, HTC, LG, and General Electric.

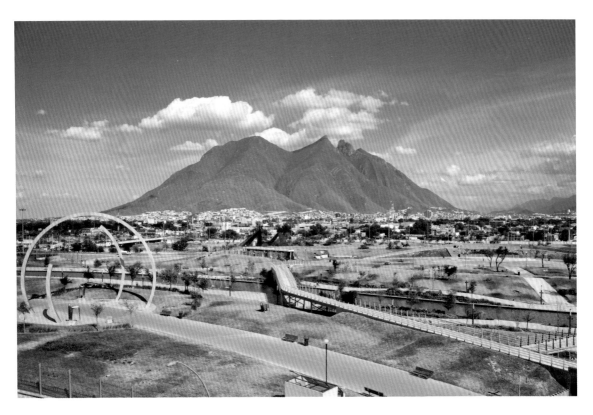

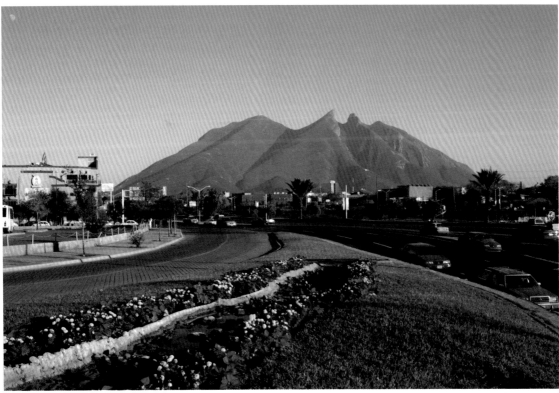

Cerro de la Silla (Saddle Mountain)

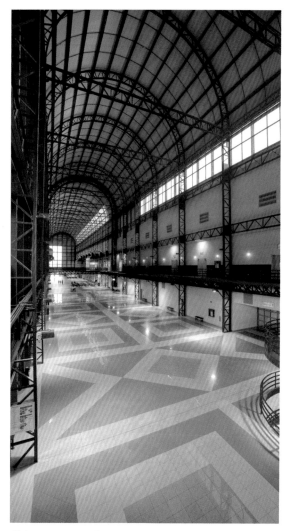

Cintermex, convention center

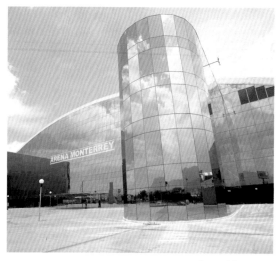

Arena Monterrey

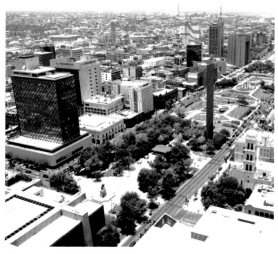

Macroplaza, downtown Monterrey

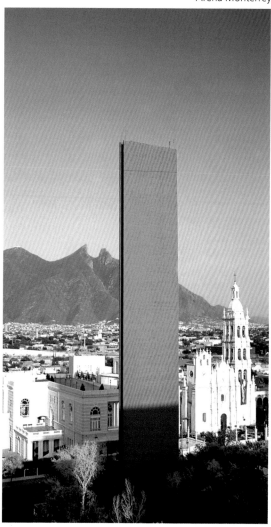

Faro del Comercio (Lighthouse of Commerce)

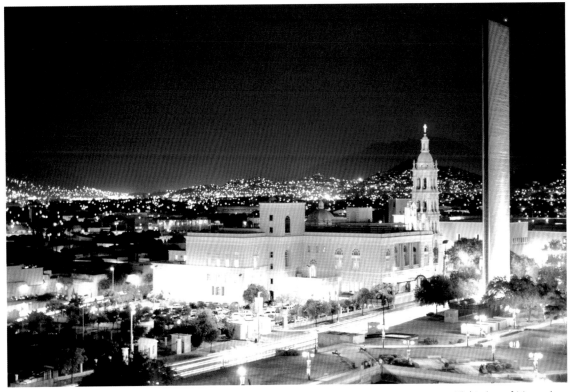

Night view of Macroplaza

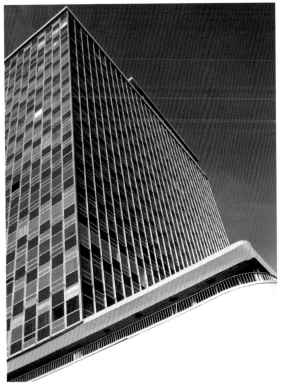

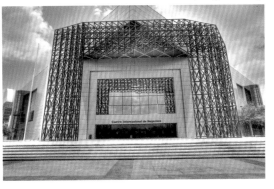

Puente de la Unidad (Bridge of Unity)

Edificio Acero (Steel Building)

Cintermex

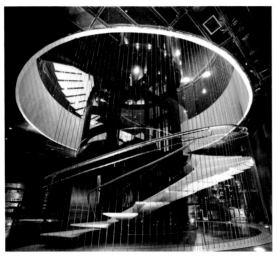

Museo del Acero Horno3 (Horno3 Steel Museum)

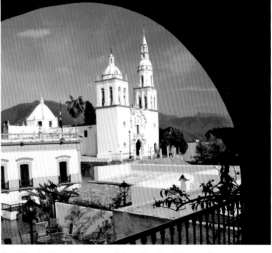

Pueblo de Santiago, a traditional, colonial-era village

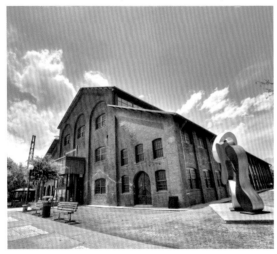

Centro de las Artes CONARTE (Center of the Arts)

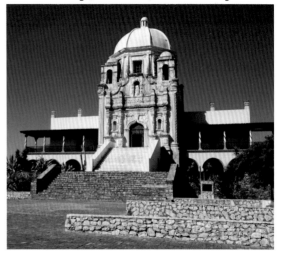

Palacio del Obispado (Bishop's Palace)

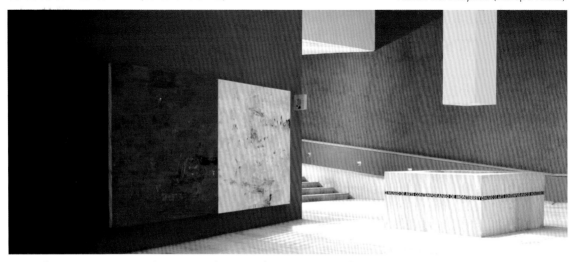

Museo de Arte Contemporáneo de Monterrey (Museum of Contemporary Art)

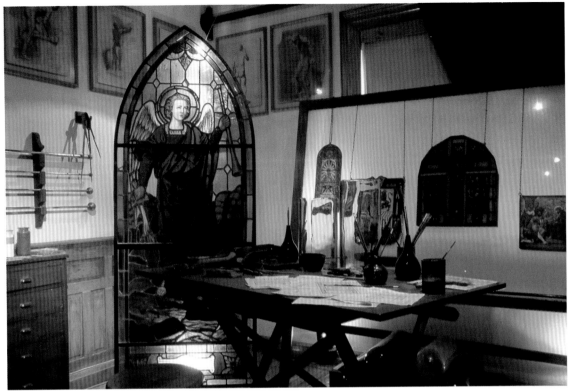

Museo del Vidrio (Glass Museum)

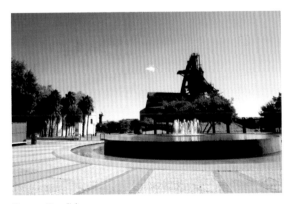

Parque Fundidora

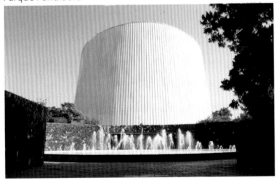

Planetario Alfa, a planetarium and IMAX dome

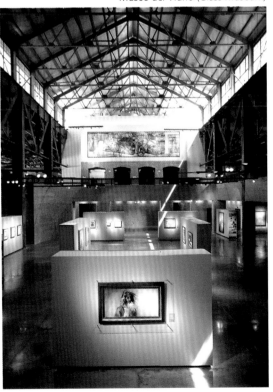

Center of the Arts

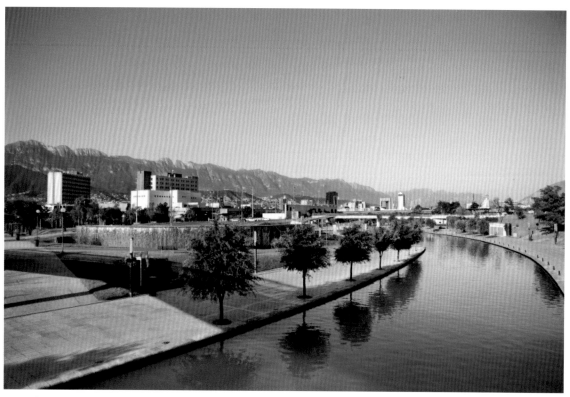

Paseo de Santa Lucía (Santa Lucía Riverwalk)

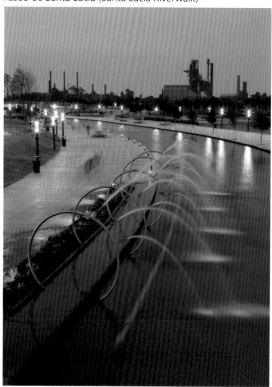

Santa Lucía Riverwalk

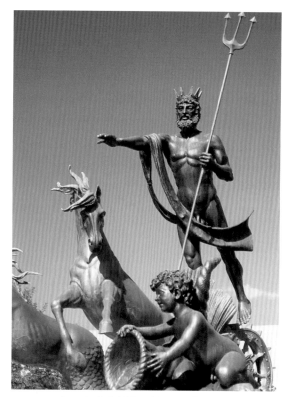

Fuente de la Vida o Neptuno (Neptune Fountain)

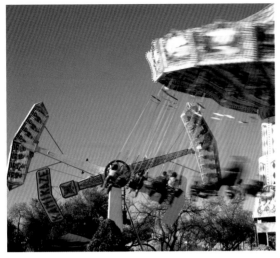

Bosque Mágico (Magic Forest), theme park

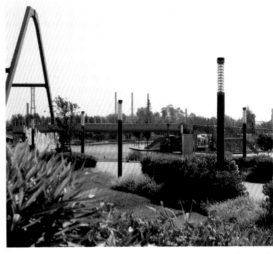

Santa Lucía Riverwalk

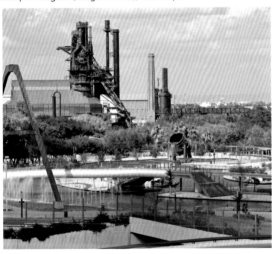

Santa Lucía Riverwalk

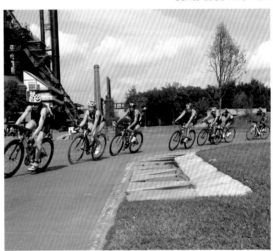

2011 Monterrey ITU Triathlon World Cup

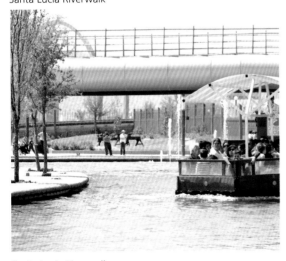

Santa Lucía Riverwalk

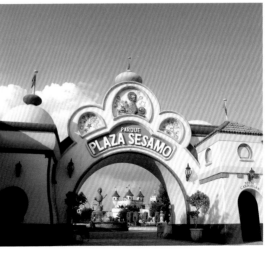

Parque Plaza Sésamo (Sesame Street Amusement Park)

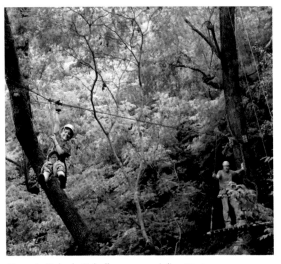

Cascada Cola de Caballo, canopy zipline tour

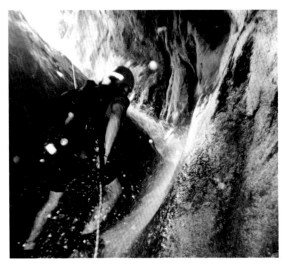

Matacanes Canyon

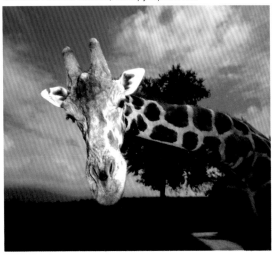

Bioparque Estrella, wildlife park

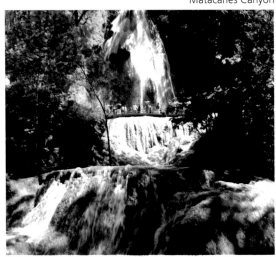

Cascada Cola de Caballo (Horsetail Falls)

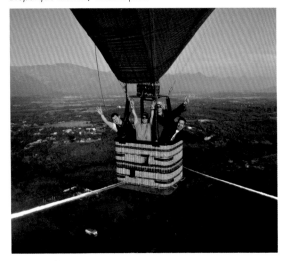

Balloon ride over Monterrey

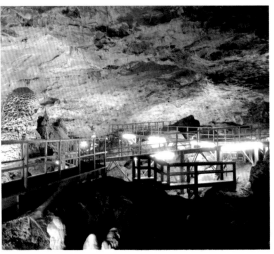

Grutas de Garcia (García Caves)

The Medical Traveler's Essentials for Monterrey, Mexico

This section provides a handy rundown of practical information on transportation, currency, communications, and other "nuts and bolts" of travel to Mexico.

Note: Regulations and procedures for travel to Mexico vary depending on the country of origin, destination, citizenship, length of stay, and more. *The following information applies to US citizens only.* Medical travelers from other countries should check with their in-nation passport offices and officials at the Mexican embassy.

Passport/Passport Card

All US citizens, including children, must present a valid passport or passport card for travel to and from Mexico. US legal permanent residents in possession of an I-551 Permanent Resident Card may board flights to the US from Mexico. As of May 1, 2010, non-US citizens with valid US visas may enter Mexico and do not have to obtain a Mexican visa.

The US Passport Card has been in full production since July 2008. As of March 1, 2010, Mexican immigration accepts the passport card for entry into Mexico by air; however, the card may not be used to board international flights in the US or to return to the US from abroad by air. The card is available only to US citizens and is primarily intended for residents who cross the border frequently by land.

The US Department of State strongly encourages all American citizen travelers to apply for a US passport well in advance of anticipated travel. American citizens can visit the Bureau of Consular Affairs website (travel.state.gov) or call 1 877 4USA.PPT (487.2778) for information on applying for passports. Many post offices in the US can also take passport applications.

Minors

Mexican law requires that any non-Mexican citizen under the age of 18 departing Mexico carry a notarized written permission from any parent or guardian not traveling with the child to or from Mexico. This permission must include the name of the parent, the name of the child, the name of anyone traveling with the child, and the notarized signature(s) of the absent parent(s). The US State Department recommends that the written permission include travel dates, destinations, airlines, and a brief summary of the circumstances surrounding the travel. The child must carry the original letter (not a facsimile or scanned copy) as well as proof of the parent/child relationship (usually a birth certificate or court document) and an original custody decree, if applicable. Travelers should contact the Mexican embassy or the nearest Mexican consulate for current information.

Tourist Cards

If you're flying or driving to Monterrey, you must pay a fee to obtain a tourist card or Forma Migratoria Múltiple (FMM), which is available from

Mexican consulates, Mexican border crossing points, Mexican tourism offices, airports within the border zone, and most airlines serving Mexico.

The fee for the tourist card is generally included in the price of a plane ticket. US citizens fill out the FMM form; Mexican immigration retains the large portion of the form and the traveler is given the smaller portion. The FMM is normally white, blue, and green. It is extremely important to keep the form in a safe location. Upon exiting the country at a Mexican immigration departure checkpoint, US citizens are required to turn in this form.

The US Department of State is aware of cases in which US citizens without their FMM have been required to change their flight (at personal expense), file a police report with local authorities regarding the missing document, and visit an Instituto Nacional de Migración (INM) office to pay a fine and obtain a valid exit visa. In other cases, travelers have been able to continue their journey after paying a fine. It's not worth gambling on: don't lose the document!

Smart Traveler Enrollment Program

US citizens living or traveling in Mexico are encouraged to sign up for the Smart Traveler Enrollment Program, either online at travelregistration .state.gov or directly with the nearest US embassy or consulate. Enrolling is important; it allows the State Department to assist US citizens in an emergency and keep them up to date with important safety and security announcements.

US Consulate, Monterrey
Avenida Constitución #411 Pte.
Monterrey, Nuevo León, MEXICO 64000
Tel: +52 81 8047.3100; +52 81 8362.9126 for after-hours emergencies
Email: monterreyACS@state.gov
Web: monterrey.usconsulate.gov

Immunizations

The US Department of State does not currently list any HIV/AIDS entry restrictions for visitors to, or foreign residents in, Mexico. The US Centers for Disease Control and Prevention (CDC) recommends routine immunizations for all travelers. Hepatitis A immunization is also recommended for travelers to Mexico. The typhoid vaccine is recommended for all unvaccinated people traveling to Mexico and Central America, especially if staying with friends or relatives or visiting smaller cities, villages, or rural areas where exposure might occur through food or water. To get the most benefit from your vaccines, see a healthcare provider at least 4–6 weeks before your trip. Visit the CDC's website at cdc.gov/travel for its latest travel health guidelines.

Health

Traveler's diarrhea is the most common travel-related ailment. Most cases of traveler's diarrhea are mild and do not require either antibiotics or antidiarrheal drugs. Adequate fluid intake is *essential*. If diarrhea is severe or bloody, or if fever occurs with shaking chills, or if abdominal pain becomes marked, or if diarrhea persists for more than 72 hours, medical attention should be sought.

The best way to prevent diarrhea is to be very careful about the water you drink. In most hotels and restaurants, you will be served purified water. If in doubt, ask for it: "*Agua purificada, por favor.*" Refrain from drinking water from the tap in a private home or condominium, just to be on the safe side. Buy bottled water, and drink a lot of it.

Though effective, antibiotics are not recommended prophylactically (i.e., to prevent diarrhea before it occurs) because of the risk of adverse side effects, though this approach may be warranted in special situations, such as for immunocompromised travelers.

Customs Regulations

US citizens bringing gifts to friends and relatives in Mexico should be prepared to demonstrate to Mexican customs officials the origin and value of the gifts. US citizens entering Mexico by land borders can bring in gifts with a value of up to US$75 duty-free, except for alcohol and tobacco products. US citizens entering Mexico by air or sea can bring in gifts with a value of up to US$300 duty-free.

Tourists are allowed to bring in their personal effects duty-free. According to customs regulations, in addition to clothing, personal effects may include

- one camera
- one video camera
- one personal computer
- five DVDs
- one mobile phone

If you are carrying these items, even if they're duty-free, you should enter the "merchandise to declare" lane at the first customs checkpoint and be prepared to pay any assessed duty. Failure to declare personal effects can result in the seizure of the goods as contraband.

Getting Help

- Police: 066
- Medical emergencies: 065
- Fire: 068
- General emergencies: 066; 911 is redirected to 066 in larger cities
- US Consulate, Monterrey: +52 81 8047.3100; +52 81 8362.9126 for after-hours emergencies

Credit Cards and ATMs

All major credit cards except Discover are widely accepted throughout Monterrey. In smaller restaurants, it's best to ask before ordering: not every business takes credit cards. Banks give cash advances on credit cards, and most of them have ATM machines for after-hours cash. Most of the malls and shopping areas have banks or ATMs where travelers can obtain cash if needed.

Electrical Appliances

If you are from the US or Canada, your small appliances (hair dryer, toothbrush, and the like) will all work. Mexico uses standard plug types A and B at 120V, the same voltage as the rest of North America. If you're coming from Europe, or any country that uses 220 volts, you'll need the proper adapters.

Mobile Phone Use

Monterrey has reliable telecommunications services which should be hassle-free for any traveler. If you plan to bring your own mobile phone, be sure to check with your provider about international service rates for voice and data. Be especially careful if you have data services on your mobile phone since automated data services can lead to shocking, unwelcome billing surprises when you get home!

If you really need mobile service in Monterrey, it might be easier and cheaper to take advantage of one of the many prepaid mobile promotions that include a mobile and a preset number of minutes. You will then have a phone whenever you travel in Monterrey. Representatives from Telcel, Mexico's largest telecommunications provider, can handle any inquiries about service usage and international connections at telcel.com and look for the "traveling to Mexico" link.

Attractions and Accommodations in Monterrey, Mexico

———————————————————————

W hatever you're thinking about seeing, doing, or experiencing outside of your hospital stay, chances are good that you'll find it in Monterrey. If you're interested in history, museums, and cultural activities, there's more than enough here to fill your free time, including wonderful restaurants, vibrant nightlife, and excellent shopping opportunities. Hiking, riding, and climbing are all available just outside Monterrey, and the surrounding mountains, canyons, and deserts are famous for their beauty and richness. Be sure to bring a camera!

Most of the hotels are located in an area known as the Centro de Monterrey. It's a lively square within walking distance of the Macroplaza, which comprises a park, an outdoor bazaar, and cafés that feature Mexican music and dancers on the weekends.

Information on Tourism and Local Events

For maps and local event listings, visit Monterrey's official tourism center, the Infotur Tourist Office, on the third floor of the Elizando Paez Building located at 5 de Mayo 525 Ote, near the north end of the Macroplaza. The office is open from 9 a.m. to 7:30 p.m. and keeps a current listing of most attractions, including theater performances, concerts, art exhibitions, cultural events, and sporting events. It also has the best supply of maps and brochures in the city. You can reach the office by telephone at +52 81 8345.0870.

Staying Safe in Monterrey

In recent years, stories of drug-cartel violence in Mexico have become increasingly common. Is Monterrey safe for a visitor? Yes, if you use your head and follow the new rules of the road. Trust only established providers of travel arrangements, and don't head off on your own. Don't rent cars or take your own tours. Use only official taxis. Use guides and tour leaders recommended by your hospital's international patient staff. Stay in a major international hotel and ask the concierge there to arrange transportation and sightseeing for you.

As you would do anywhere, especially in any urban area, beware of walking alone on dark streets at night. Don't wear flashy jewelry or carry large sums of cash. If possible, walk in pairs and stick to busy, lighted areas of the city. Most restaurants will be happy to call a taxi for you if asked. This may take a little more time than hailing one on the street, but it is generally safer. Monterrey is as safe as you make it. With reasonable care, your chances of problems are no greater than in any other big city.

On the flip side, make sure your own behavior is exemplary. Be aware that Mexican authorities can fine or incarcerate those who do not follow Mexican laws. Don't jeopardize your trip by taking foolish risks. Stay smart and stay safe!

Getting Into and Around Town

By Land. Those who choose to drive from the US to Monterrey via free and toll highways need only about 2 hours' travel time from the border with Texas via Laredo (140 miles, 225 kilometers) and 3 hours from McAllen, Texas (150 miles, 240 kilometers). Distances from other major US cities: San Antonio, Texas: 305 miles, 490 kilometers; Houston, Texas: 491 miles, 790 kilometers.

By Air. You can fly to Monterrey from large US cities, and all major cities in Mexico offer direct flights to Monterrey. Monterrey's main airport is located about 10 miles (16 kilometers) north of the city (or a half hour from the hotel district). The airport has an ATM for travelers who wish to convert money right away. (Always use the ATM; the exchange offices offer a less favorable conversion rate.)

Shuttles and taxis are available at the airport, although most medical travelers already have their transportation arranged in advance with a medical travel agency or with their hospital. If yours is not arranged for you, you can and should book your airport transfer in advance. Airport transfer is offered in a choice of either standard or VIP services. Standard shuttles will transport up to ten people and their baggage in a comfortable van to and from local hotels; the VIP option provides transportation exclusively for your party, taking you and your belongings directly to and from your local hotel.

Taxis. Once you are situated in Centro de Monterrey, you should need little in the way of motorized transport: lots of what you'll want to see and do is within walking distance of the city center. Still, taxis are readily available; ask your hotel to call one for you, as that's safer and more reliable than looking for one yourself. Hotel-summoned-cab rates are usually higher than those for cabs you hail on the street, but the added safety is worth the extra cost. Monterrey's taxis are metered, but if you speak Spanish, you will enjoy a distinct advantage in your negotiations with local taxi drivers.

Dining and Nightlife

Monterrey's Barrio Antiguo or "old city" is concentrated on two main streets and a couple of side streets; it's truly the heartbeat of the city's nightlife. It offers huge dance clubs, myriad restaurants, and some very cool bars. Cars drive back and forth in this area, their occupants seeking to notice and be noticed, while hundreds of people stroll the streets for the same reasons. It's fun just to people-watch!

While many international restaurants serve simple wine-and-cheese offerings to tourists, others specialize in traditional fare. In Monterrey, that's goat. *Cabrito* is kid goat (roughly the equivalent of veal) that's been cooked on embers. It's a recipe based on Jewish cuisine. The families that settled Monterrey with Diego de Montemayor had Jewish origins, and the city has stayed faithful to them.

You can taste those same origins in *semita*, which is unleavened bread, and *capirotada*, a dessert made of cooked bread, cheese, raisins, peanuts, and crystallized sugarcane juice. And goats return to the menu at dessert time: their milk is used in the traditional Monterrey candies known as *glorias* and *obleas*.

Shredded beef with eggs is *machacado con huevo*. *Carne asada*—the Mexican equivalent of barbecued beef—is also popular. The latter appears in a number of different dishes, from tacos to combination dinners of *carne asada*, baked potatoes, sausages, and grilled onions.

Monterrey has a long history of supporting local breweries, and the beer is delicious! Clubs are quiet until midnight and are open until four o'clock in the morning, so you need to be a real night owl to spend time there! The drinking age is 18, though inspection of age identification isn't widely enforced. Weekends are the most crowded, while Sunday evenings and early weekdays can be slow.

Tipping

Tipping in Mexico follows the guidelines familiar to most travelers in the Americas: 10–15 percent for restaurant servers and hotel staff, and US$1–$2 per bag for porters who carry luggage. You may want to tip nursing and service staff in hospitals if you feel you received excellent service.

Things to do in Monterrey

1. Take a walk through the **Parque Niños Héroes** and visit the art gallery, science museum, and botanical garden. There's even a terrific glass-domed aviary featuring hundreds of bird species!

2. Soak up Nuevo León's artistic heritage at the galleries of **La Pinacoteca del Estado**.

3. Check out the **Cervecería Cuauhtémoc-Moctezuma**—the oldest brewery in Monterrey, now a museum—before heading to a café to sample some of the local brews.

4. Even if you're not Catholic, the **Capilla de los Dulces Nombres** is worth a visit if you'd like a little quiet time. In the Macroplaza, you can also visit the **Catedral Metropolitana de Nuestra Señora de Monterrey**, which took 150 years to complete.

5. Visit the **Parque Nacional Cumbres de Monterrey**, where hiking trails wind through the mountains and provide visitors with a pleasant getaway from the metropolis. The easiest walk is Chipinque, on the southwestern edge of town, and a good choice for post-surgery!

6. Stroll through the **Barrio Antiguo** and look in all the windows of the antique and specialty shops you pass; sit in a café with a strong coffee when you start to get tired. In September the cultural and folkloric Festival Internacional de Santa Lucía is held here.

7. Take the kids to the **Parque Plaza Sésamo**, an amusement park featuring many high-technology attractions.

8. Go (slightly) out of town to visit the **Pueblo de Santiago**, a town with cobbled streets, colonial buildings, and some of the best restaurants in Monterrey.

9. Have your hotel pack you a picnic and head up to the **Cascada Cola de Caballo** to enjoy it. (Do you think the waterfall really looks like a horse's tail?)

10. Take a ride through the **Bioparque Estrella**, a wildlife park that features a drive-through safari and a children's petting zoo. ∎

Other Local Attractions and Landmarks

- The Paseo Santa Lucía (Santa Lucía Riverwalk), a lovely artificial river built between 1996 and 2007
- The Cerro de la Silla (Saddle Mountain)
- The Macroplaza, the cultural and administrative heart of the city, featuring remarkable monuments and green areas and surrounded by many of Monterrey's most famous buildings
- The Faro del Comercio (Lighthouse of Commerce), another landmark of the city, which beams a green laser around the city at night
- The Museo de Arte Contemporáneo de Monterrey (Museum of Modern Art), with its post-modern Mexican architecture designed by Ricardo Legorreta
- Monterrey's Inukshuk, one of only a handful of authentic examples to be found outside Canada of these stone monuments from the high Arctic
- The Parque Fundidora, a large urban park that contains old foundry buildings, nearly 300 acres (120 hectares) of natural ambiance, artificial lakes, playgrounds, an alternative cinema (the Cineteca), and a museum (photo collection, state plastic arts collection, and other exhibits), plus a hotel, auditorium, and convention center
- The Puente de la Unidad (Bridge of Unity), a suspension bridge that crosses Río Santa Catarina and joins San Pedro Garza García with Monterrey
- The Planetario Alfa, a planetarium with the first IMAX dome built in Latin America (the fourth in the world)
- The Palacio de Gobierno, a pink marble structure of neoclassical architecture where the governor's office is located
- The Cerro del Obispado (Bishopric Hill), topped by a scenic lookout called Mirador del Obispado, and featuring a museum inside the Palacio del Obispado (Bishop's Palace)

- Two distinctive buildings at Instituto Tecnológico: CEDES, which houses the institute's nationwide administration; and CETEC, which houses the main computer classroom and other offices
- The Salón de la Fama (Baseball Hall of Fame) at the Cervecería Cuauhtémoc-Moctezuma brewery

Shopping

Monterrey offers unique shopping experiences, including everything from US-style malls to quaint handicraft shops. The Zona Rosa in the *centro historico* is a popular shopping street. The two main markets in downtown Monterrey are the Mercado Juárez and the Mercado Colón. Both sell a mixture of everyday goods, collectibles, clothing, and gifts. Bargaining is definitely permissible.

South of the city, the busy roadside shopping area of Los Cavazos offers clay pots and dishes, leather products, wooden toys, musical instruments, and much more. The Mercado de Artesanías (handicraft market) features a variety of crafts, ranging from beautiful hand-painted pottery to hand-woven baskets and hammocks.

The Galerías Valle Oriente is one of the newest and most modern fashion malls in Monterrey. The US-style Galerías Monterrey hosts a variety of department stores, a food court, specialty shops, and modern technology, offering name brands for less. The Plaza Fiesta San Agustín is a mall that blends department stores with popular coffee shops. The glass-domed Plaza México, located in the heart of Monterrey, contains more than a hundred stores and restaurants.

Where to Stay

Monterrey has more than 8,500 hotel rooms! Check with your medical travel agency or hospital to find one that meets your personal preferences and provides easy access to your chosen healthcare facility. Also, be sure to ask about discounts when you make your reservation. Discounts are often available for extended stays, and some hospitals have negotiated rates.

Hotels: Deluxe

Presidente Monterrey	Avenida José Vasconcelos #300 Ote. San Pedro Garza García Monterrey, Nuevo León, MEXICO 66260 Tel: +52 81 8368.6000 Email: shpresidente@hotelesmilenium.com Web: ichotelsgroup.com
Safi Royal Luxury	Avenida Diego Rivera #555 Colonia Valle Oriente Monterrey, Nuevo León, MEXICO 66260 Tel: +52 81 8100.7080 Email: reservacionesvalle@safihotel.com Web: www.safihotel.com
Sheraton Ambassador	Avenida Hidalgo #310 Colonia Valle Oriente Monterrey, Nuevo León, MEXICO 64000 Tel: +52 81 8380.7000 Email: monterrey.sheraton@sheraton.com Web: starwoodhotels.com
Crown Plaza Hotel Monterrey	Avenida Constitución #300 Oriente Colonia Centro Monterrey, Nuevo León, MEXICO 64000 Tel: +52 81 8319.6000; 1 877 227.6963, US toll-free Email: ventas_cpm@hotelesmilenium.com Web: ichotelsgroup.com
Quinta Real Monterrey	Avenida Diego Rivera #500 Colonia Centro Monterrey, Nuevo León, MEXICO 66260 Tel: +1 52 55 1105.1000; 1 866 621.9288, US toll-free Web: quintarealhotels.com
Hotel Chipinque	Meseta de Chipinque #1000 San Pedro Garza García Monterrey, Nuevo León, MEXICO 67320 Tel: +52 81 8173.1777 Email: ventas@hotelchipinque.com Web: hotelchipinque.com
Hotel Hacienda Cola de Caballo	Carretera a Cola de Caballo Km 6 El Cercado Santiago, Nuevo León, MEXICO 67320 Tel: +52 81 2285.0660 Email: hotel@coladecaballo.com Web: coladecaballo.com/ingles

Hotels: Moderate

Fiesta Inn Monterrey Valle	Avenida Lázaro Cárdenas #427 Ote. San Pedro Garza García Monterrey, Nuevo León, MEXICO 66269 Tel: +52 81 8399.1500; 1 800 343.7821, US toll-free Web: fiestainn.com
Wyndham Casa Grande Monterrey	Avenida Lázaro Cárdenas #2305 Residencial San Agustín San Pedro Garza García, Nuevo León, MEXICO 66260 Tel: +52 81 8133.0808 Web: wyndham.com
Hampton Inn Monterrey– Galerias Obispado Hotel	Avenida Gonzalitos #415 Sur Obispado Monterrey, Nuevo León, MEXICO 64060 Tel: +52 81 8625.2450 Web: hamptoninn.com
Holiday Inn Express San Jerónimo	Avenida San Jerónimo #1082 Colonia San Jerónimo Monterrey, Nuevo León, MEXICO 64640 Tel: +52 81 8389.6000 Email: ventas_hiegal@hotelesmilenium.com Web: hiexpress.com
Hotel Misión Monterrey Centro	Fray Servando Padre Mier #201 Monterrey, Nuevo León, MEXICO 64000 Tel: +52 81 8150.6500 Web: hotelesmision.com

Wherever you choose to stay, you can be sure that Mexico's famous warmth and hospitality will embrace you and make you feel comfortable from the moment you arrive until your day of departure. If you have any further questions about hotels, feel free to ask your medical travel agency or your hospital for recommendations. Staff members there will be glad to help.

Part Four

Resources and References

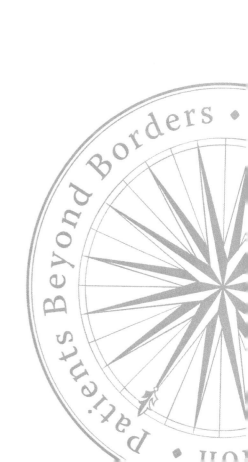

Additional Resources

World, Country, and City Information

The World Factbook. Cataloged by country, *The World Factbook*—compiled by the US Central Intelligence Agency (CIA)—is an excellent source of general, up-to-date information about the geography, economy, and history of countries around the world. Go to cia.gov; in the left column, find "Library," then click "Publications." *Factbook* lets you explore places of interest by region and country.

Lonely Planet. This feisty travel book publisher has compiled a collection of useful online snippets (mostly as teasers to get you to buy its books), along with useful links. Go to lonelyplanet.com for an introduction to Monterrey, links to Monterrey blogs, and an option to buy PDF chapters from Lonely Planet's latest Mexico edition.

World Travel Guide. The publishers of the *Columbus World Travel Guide* sponsor worldtravelguide.net. Go to the website and choose a continent to find information on countries, cities, airports, cruise destinations, and more.

Wikitravel. This consumer-contributed, grassroots project—wikitravel. org—intends to create a free, complete, up-to-date, and reliable worldwide travel guide. The site collects destination guides and other articles written and edited by travelers around the globe. On the home page you'll find recommendations for the "Destination of the Month" and some fascinating factoids about exotic locations. Click on a continent or region for more information, Wiki-style.

CDC Travel. The US Centers for Disease Control and Prevention (CDC) maintains a guide for traveler's health at cdc.gov/travel. The site provides health information on more than 200 international destinations, as well as general information about vaccinations and alerts about disease outbreaks and other health hazards. A useful "Find a Clinic" link leads to travel health specialists and yellow fever vaccination clinics.

One World Nations Online. For everything you ever wanted to know about Mexico, check out nationsonline.org/oneworld/mexico.htm. There you'll find links to official Mexican government websites, weather forecasts, maps, news, and all the country's major tourist attractions.

Passports and Visas

US State Department, Bureau of Consular Affairs. The website travel. state.gov connects you with the agency that oversees visas and passports into and out of the US. Country-specific information, travel alerts, and travel warnings are also available on this site.

Travisa. Dozens of online agencies offer visa services. We've found Travisa, at travisa.com, to be reliable and accessible by telephone as well as internet. The agency offers good customer service and followup. Travisa's website also carries links to immunization requirements, travel warnings, current weather, and more.

Tools from *Patients Beyond Borders*

Publications

Healthy Travel Media publishes the international edition of *Patients Beyond Borders* (PBB) as well as a variety of specialized editions covering destinations from Singapore to Turkey. Visit patientsbeyondborders.com to check on special editions for your destination.

Online and Mobile Applications

Patient referral website. The *Patients Beyond Borders* technology and editorial teams have converted PBB's library of global healthcare information into consumer-focused digital products. PBB's consumer database allows patients to research and connect with healthcare providers worldwide; it offers searchable information on top country destinations, leading facilities and specialty centers, medical travel-friendly specialties and procedures, selected health travel facilitators, and patient stories. Visit patientsbeyondborders.com.

Patient referral service. Call us and we'll help match you with a provider or facility that can meet your needs. We can match your preferences for costs, location, specialty, treatment, and more. Visit patientsbeyondborders.com for more information or call: 1 800 883.5740, US toll-free, +1 919 924.0636, international.

TravelEmergency. The TravelEmergency® mobile application allows users to access emergency health resources in top tourist destinations. Application resources include destination-specific emergency numbers, listings for top medical facilities (with emergency contact information), a phrase-finder with common phrases translated into ten languages, and an emergency alert feature for friends and family. Learn more at patientsbeyondborders.com/travel-emergency. ■

Currency Converter

xe.com. To learn quickly how much your money is worth in your country of interest, go to xe.com and use the "Universal Currency Converter." The site also provides services for money transfers and foreign payments. There's even a mobile app showing real-time currency rates for the iPhone, BlackBerry, Android, and other smartphones.

International Hospital Accreditation

Joint Commission International (JCI). Mentioned frequently throughout this book, JCI remains the only game in town for international hospital accreditation. For a current list of accredited hospitals by country, go to jointcommissioninternational.org.

International Calls

Country Calling Codes. Quickly find dialing codes from anywhere to anywhere—there's even a reverse directory that tells you the country if all you know is the code. Check it out at countrycallingcodes.com.

Skype. Get Skype on your laptop from skype.com and start talking face-to-face with other Skype users. One-to-one video calls and instant messaging are free. Skype also offers premium rates on long-distance mobile-phone calling; and a small fee monthly covers group video calls. There's a mobile app, too (see sidebar).

Mobile Applications

GoogleTranslate. This free reference app for the iPhone and iPod touch translates words and phrases between more than 50 languages. For most languages, you can speak your phrases and hear the corresponding translations.

Skype mobile. Call, video call, and instant message any other Skype user.

Google Maps. Get driving, transit, biking, or walking directions in a list or on a map. Search for businesses—even find out where your friends are. Most features work with any smartphone.

OnTheFly. This app from ITA allows you to compare air travel options across airlines, dates, and alternate cities and airports. It finds available flights with optimal fares using Android, BlackBerry, iPhone, iPod touch, or other mobile devices.

TripIt. TripIt's free apps keep your itineraries at the ready on your smartphone. They let you instantly access all the information you might need on the road, even when you can't connect to the Internet. Several other useful TripIt apps are available for iPhone, Android, and BlackBerry.

Medical Information

MedlinePlus. This US government–sponsored website brings together a wealth of information from sources such as the National Library of Medicine (the world's largest medical library), the National Institutes of Health, *Merriam-Webster's Medical Dictionary*, and the *United States Pharmacopeia*. Go to medlineplus.gov and choose "Health Topics," "Drugs and Supplements," or "Videos and Cool Tools." Sign up for email alerts or download the mobile version.

Mayo Clinic Health Information. At mayoclinic.com/health-information, more than 3,300 physicians, scientists, and researchers from the Mayo Clinic share their expertise to empower consumers and patients to manage their health. Users can search by symptoms, diseases and conditions, drugs, supplements, tests, procedures, and much more.

WebMD. The award-winning site webmd.com offers credible and in-depth medical news, features, reference material, and online community programs. Search alphabetically or by categories, including drugs, supplements, conditions, and parenting. There are even sections on pet health and teen health. Sign up for newsletters that deliver everything from cholesterol management advice to a healthy recipe daily.

Medical Travel Resources

International Medical Travel Journal (IMTJ). *IMTJ* is the world's leading journal for the medical travel industry. While geared more toward industry professionals than consumers, it does provide a free downloadable guide for patients at imtjonline.com. There's a free email newsletter, too, and a comprehensive directory of medical tourism companies, agencies, hospitals, clinics, doctors, and dentists who specialize in treating international patients.

Medical Travel Today. This free newsletter of the medical tourism industry reports trends, deals, new business, competition, medical advances, legal issues, and the advancement of care for the rapidly growing ranks of medical travelers. It is published twice monthly and emailed to subscribers. Sign up at medical traveltoday.com.

International Society of Travel Medicine (ISTM). If you are looking for information about immunizations, infectious diseases, or other aspects of medical travel, check out the ISTM website, istm.org. This organization (headquartered in Decatur, Georgia) seeks to promote safe and healthy travel and to facilitate education, service, and research activities in the field of travel medicine. Most useful to the global patient is the society's searchable database of health travel practitioners.

Medeguide. This online doctor-finder service features and profiles hundreds of international physicians, primarily those working in affiliation with large, internationally accredited hospitals. Medeguide's information is provided by the doctors themselves or by the hospitals where they work. Patients can search for doctors by country, hospital, specialty, procedure, or condition. Learn more at medeguide.com.

Index

Specific treatments are in *italics*. Hospital names and specialist groups are in **bold**. Main treatment categories are indexed; specific treatments may be found in the text.

ABOUT THE AUTHOR

As president of Healthy Travel Media and author of *Patients Beyond Borders*, **Josef Woodman** has spent more than five years touring 150 medical facilities in 30 countries, researching international healthcare travel. Cofounder of MyDailyHealth and Ventana Communications, Woodman's pioneering background in health, publishing, and web technology has allowed him to compile a wealth of information about global health travel, telemedicine, and consumer-directed healthcare demand.

Woodman has lectured at the UCLA School of Public Health, Harvard Medical School, and Duke Fuqua School of Business, and has chaired and keynoted conferences on medical tourism and global healthcare in 14 countries. He has appeared in numerous print and broadcast media, including CNN, ABC News, Fox News, *The New York Times*, *Barron's*, *The Wall Street Journal*, and more. Woodman is an outspoken advocate of affordable, high-quality medical care for healthcare consumers worldwide.